Cover and book design by Danielle Larsen "The magic gal with the mouse"

Special thanks to my copy editor, Nancy Wall.

Order this book online at www.trafford.com
or email orders@trafford.com

Most Trafford titles are also available at major online book retailers.

© Copyright 2010 J. Warren Willey II.
All rights reserved. No part of this publication may be reproduced, stored in a retrieval system, or transmitted, in any form or by any means, electronic, mechanical, photocopying, recording, or otherwise, without the written prior permission of the author.

Printed in Victoria, BC, Canada.

ISBN: 978-1-4269-3038-6 (soft)
ISBN: 978-1-4269-3039-3 (hard)

Library of Congress Control Number: 2010905552

Our mission is to efficiently provide the world's finest, most comprehensive book publishing service, enabling every author to experience success. To find out how to publish your book, your way, and have it available worldwide, visit us online at www.trafford.com

Trafford rev. 7/15/2010

Trafford Publishing® www.trafford.com

North America & international
toll-free: 1 888 232 4444 (USA & Canada)
phone: 250 383 6864 ♦ fax: 812 355 4082

This book is not intended to replace medical advice. Nothing can compare to a face-to-face conversation with your doctor with regards to your health. If you are sick, or suspect you are sick, you need to see your doctor. If you are taking prescription medication, talk to your health care provider before making dietary changes, as the metabolism of the drugs you are on may be affected. Talk to your doctor before starting an exercise program. It is also essential that you talk to your doctor about any supplements you may be taking, or plan to start taking after reading this book. Supplements, as well as food, can change the way your body interacts with drugs.

This book is about the power of food and *how* you can maintain weight loss for life. The author and publisher expressly disclaim responsibility for any adverse affects arising from opinions following herein.

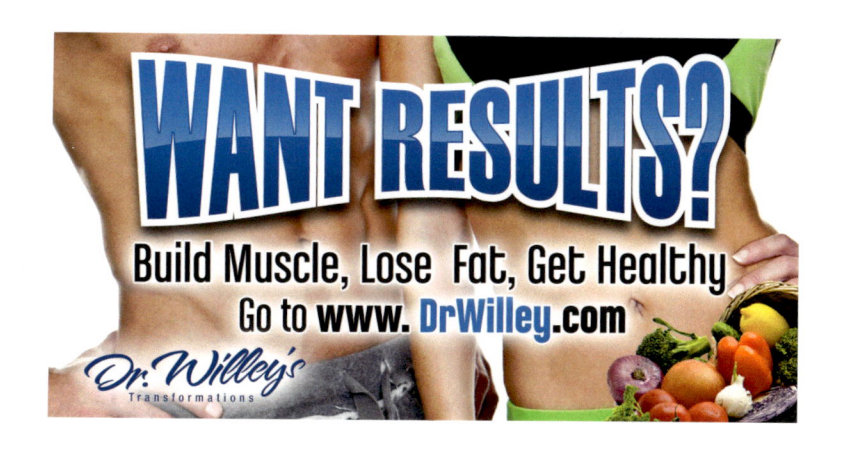

WANT RESULTS?
Build Muscle, Lose Fat, Get Healthy
Go to www.DrWilley.com

Dr. Willey's Transformations

Dedication

*The **Z** Diet is dedicated to my three children. They are my gift from God. They are my reason for living, my excuse for playing, and my realization that there is so much more to life than what I see. I love you three so much - you little turkeys! I must also give all credit to GOD, as nothing is possible without him, and everything is possible through him.*

*The best of health and **Z**ellness!*

Part 1
Chapter 1 - **Introduction**
    Why short term weight loss programs do not work – adherence
    The Law of Free Money

Part 2 – Your Starting Point
Chapter 2 - Body Category Designation
    Metabolically challenged
        Insulin
    Hormonally challenged
    Physique Oriented
    General health
Chapter 3 - **The Basics of Food**
Chapter 4 - **Willey Principle**

Part 3 - What Happens when you Diet?
Chapter 5 - **Understanding Dieting**
Chapter 6 - **Quick Weight Loss Approaches**
    Diuresis
    Fasts
    VLED
    LED

Part 4 - Performance of The Z Diet
Chapter 7 - **Direct Ways to Control Calories**
    Choosing Amounts of foods
Chapter 8 - **Macro-Nutrient Breakdown**
Chapter 9 - **Subtle Ways to Control Calories – LEARN HOW TO EAT**
    Biggest meal in AM, smallest in PM
    Smaller more frequent meals vs. other
    Majority of carbs early
        Chrononutrakinetics
        Food Timing
    Don't eat before bed
    Energy OUT
    Cyclic Eating

Scheduled Breaks
Tracking Results
When Scheduled; Schedule!

Chapter 10 - **How To Shop and Read Labels**
Chapter 11 - **Medications and Weight Loss**
Chapter 12 - **Summary**
Appendix I   – The Glycemic Index
Appendix II – (Popular) Quick Weight Loss Diets
Appendix III – The Z Diet and Holidays, Parties, and Office Goodies
Appendix IV – Contact Information

1

Introduction

All diets work, whether low carb, high carb/low fat, low calorie, very low calorie, the hCG diet, or the Maple Syrup Diet. In reality, the problem in our country is not weight loss. Hundreds and thousands of pounds are lost each day. The problem is that, after they lose the weight, most people tend to turn around and find it again. Our problem is *weight loss maintenance*.

Diets, or any attempts to better one's health for that matter, come in many forms, fashions, colors, sales pitches, promises, and expenses. They even come with a variety of different delivery systems, including devices and chemicals that go up your backside...The goal with most of them is to help you get healthier, lose fat, gain strength and vitality, and better your sex life. I could go on, but you have all heard the commercials.

Let me give you a brief synopsis of almost every diet book out there – I call it the Bait, Hook, Reel You In, and Use You as Bait for the Bigger Fish - trick: It starts with a chapter or two of what I refer to as the 'warm-fuzzies'. The warm-fuzzies are soft, sweet

> **FAT FACTS**
> Percent of noninstitutionalized adults age 20 years and over who are overweight or obese: 67% and the percent of noninstitutionalized adults age 20 years and over who are obese: 34% (2005-2006)

words that rip responsibility right out from under you. "It is not your fault you are fat" or "did you know that "x" chemical in your foods is killing you?" The whole purpose is to make you feel good about what you are reading (i.e. the bait). It then convinces you that what you are about to read is the solution to your problems, in particular, your fat (that's not your fault, remember?) i.e the hook. The Reel You In portion of the book gives you a solution for weight loss that, without a doubt, works. (– mind you) This may be to cut all of your carbohydrates from your diet forever, or to remove all fat of any sort from your diet, or, better yet, remove anything from your diet that at one time walked, crawled, swam, ran, or flew! Whatever that diet book or plan's solution is, it really does work. I am not arguing that it does not. Most of these solutions work for weight loss. Once again – I said weight loss...not *weight loss maintenance!* The final strategy of these weight loss plans is the Use You as Bait for the Bigger Fish ploy: This simply throws you back in the water, so you will buy the supplements that are part of the solution, or sets you up to buy the next version of the book. It is quite beautiful, from a monetary stand point (at least for somebody...)
– but does nothing for you in the long run.

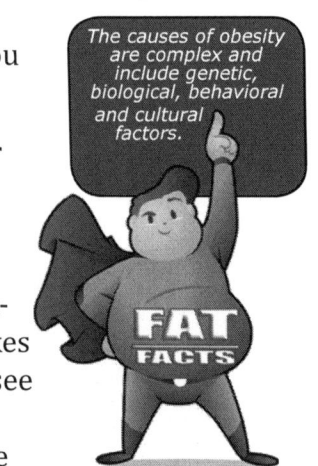

One way or another, hidden or open, subtle or obvious, trick or treat – they cut calories or have you burn more with activity. That's it. That is their secret – even if they tell you that you do not have to restrict your calories or exercise more – they get you to do it. No one likes to be limited, or told not to do something – I see no difference in my weight loss patients' attitudes toward limitation than I see in my three year old's. We hate constraint and we hate control (unless we have that control), and diet writers and diet authors know it. Their simple solution: trick you into caloric restriction or increased caloric burn by some other method. I could literally provide you with hundreds of examples, but I am sure, now that you have heard it put like this, that you can see it.

No matter what the ploy, calories come into play and are as important as can be when it comes to dieting, short term weight loss, and long term *weight loss maintenance*. There are a few situations and developed laws of weight loss that allow some variance with the calories in to calories out standard, as you will soon read, but overall – you must consider calories in weight loss – quick or slow, short or long term.

Are calories all that are important? No. The individual who participates in the diet plan comes into play. By individual, I am referring to one's psychosocial make up, emotional status, genetics, disease states, and the state of their hormones. For example, some people are more sensitive to carbohydrates and therefore do better with a weight loss plan that when restricts some of the carbohydrates - but calories will come into play.

Why short term weight loss programs don't work for long term weight loss maintenance.

I am not going to rehash everything you have ever read about the failure of dieting. We all know dieting does not really work; *really* being defined as getting to one's goals and *maintaining one's goals long term*. I am going to tell you why The Z Diet will work for you.

First, let's define *weight loss maintenance*. Maintenance is hard to define as it is largely a personal perception. Do you consider your weight loss a failure if you gain back one of ten pounds after a diet? In the world of weight loss medicine, we have a few simple

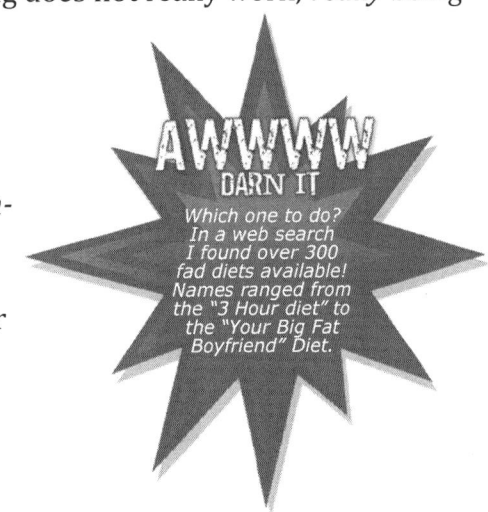

AWWWW
DARN IT
Which one to do?
In a web search
I found over 300
fad diets available!
Names ranged from
the "3 Hour diet" to
the "Your Big Fat
Boyfriend" Diet.

MEDICAL MINUTE

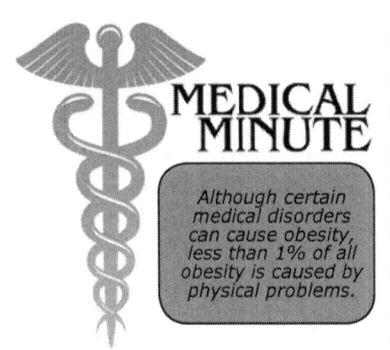

Although certain medical disorders can cause obesity, less than 1% of all obesity is caused by physical problems.

definitions: The Institute of Medicine defines *weight loss maintenance* as intentional weight loss of 5% or more, maintained for one year. The National Institute of Health defines it as weight loss of 10% or more, maintained for one year. The National Weight Control Registry considers it a weight loss of 30 pounds or more, maintained for at least one year. So who is correct? If you put real numbers into their definitions, it really is not a lot of weight. For example: according to The National Institutes of Health, if you weigh 250 pounds, and you lose 25 pounds and keep it off for a year, you are successful! Health wise, even a few pounds off your hide improves your well-being, so any fat loss is successful by my definition. As for you? Can you come up with what you would consider successful weight loss? I think it is a very personal decision, as long as it is realistic. If you dropped sixty pounds of fat from your body, but then gained thirty back, I would still consider your overall effort a success. Honestly, even if you gained fifty-nine back, you would still have succeeded.

But even with the numbers not being that substantial, why do most diets fail? And if you are able to drop a few pounds, why does your diet not work better?

In an article printed in *The American Journal of Clinical Nutrition* in February of 2007, some authors asked the same simple question: Why do obese patients not lose more weight when treated with low-calorie diets? Their answers where based on three fundamentals: 1. Fractional energy absorption; 2. Adaptations in energy expenditure; and, 3. Incomplete patient diet adherence. In English: 1. Fat people absorb more food than the rest of us; 2. Metabolism slows down when you restrict calories; and, 3. People do not follow their diets.

Let's look at each of these: 1. To my knowledge, there is no study supporting the idea that people absorb different amounts of food. Transit time may differ (how quickly food gets from point **A** to point **Brown**) but absorption rate does not. Even if larger people did "absorb more food", it could not account for the lack of weight loss on a low calorie diet, as it would not account for much. 2. I would absolutely agree that your metabolism slows down when you cut calories, but so does your use of energy. Have you ever been on a low calorie diet and felt fatigued? Did you skip the gym a few times because you were too tired to go while on a low calorie eating plan? Are you more inclined to use the elevator than the stairs while dieting? If the calories are not there (i.e. the energy is not there), your body will, in turn, lessen the energy it expends. Obviously, there is individual variance in metabolic rates from baseline and therefore it is likely safe to assume the same in the dieting state.

This brings me to a quick statement on the Set Point Theory. I bring this up because sitting with diet patients as I do every day, I hear about it. The Set Point Theory gets the credit or blame for a number of conditions I deal with. The Set Point Theory is the idea that no matter what you do in life – eat or exercise too little or too much – your body will find a weight it likes and stay there. Have nothing to eat for awhile and you will decrease your activity, then go on a mad quest for food. Once you find food, you will eat and eat until normalcy is obtained and your set point has been re-reached. There are a lot of studies on this topic in rats: starve the poor little creatures and their appetites plummet, as do their metabolism and their use of energy (sit around and watch soap operas), etc. Give them access to lots of good-tasting food and their appetites, metabolism and activity all skyrocket back up to their previous "normal". At that point, they stop engorging themselves and go about their business (likely politics...). Human studies are more difficult to interpret, but the general understanding is that our set point is a bit more screwy and dynamic at the same time. In other words, our bodies preferentially and very efficiently prefer the full fat cell vs. the empty one, i.e. they protect themselves from fat loss more than from fat gain. Unlike our politically oriented rats, we tend to go beyond our previous weight as if our bodies are protecting themselves with a little cushion (no pun intended – well maybe) in case *that* ever happens again.

I personally lean toward the 'Settling Point' of the body. This is the concept that your weight and fat levels will 'settle' at a given point, based on your environment. You surround yourself with calorie dense, sugar and fat filled snacks, and then wonder why your weight came back so easily. Exposed to great tasting, high fat, high sugar food all the time, your settling point never settles, or at least keeps going up. I will continue another discussion on the homeostatic mechanisms of our body in a coming chapter, so enough tangential mishmash. Let's continue with the study:

3. Adherence – the diet writer's best friend and worst enemy. I could write the absolutely perfect eating plan, right down to the calorie, with the perfect amount of protein, carbohydrates, and fat, and using all of your favorite foods. But if you do not stick to it, you will not lose weight. Studies have shown that, no matter what kind of diet people are on (low carb, high carb, low calorie, etc.), if they comply with the diet, they lose weight. If they do not, they do not lose weight. Simple aye? If only it were so…

Here is where The Z Diet differs: The Z Diet is a *lifestyle*. If you are reverent to the fundamentals of The Z Diet, apply the principles when appropriate, and simply make changes to your routine in the manner presented, you will be adherent to the diet. In other words, you will succeed! Adherence is perhaps the biggest obstacle in the quest for *weight loss maintenance*. Simplicity is part of the answer – hence: The Z Diet. Throughout the book I will give you a number of techniques, eating patterns, food choices, direct and indirect ways to control calories, and ways to improve your lifestyle adherence.

The Law of Free Money

One more quick qualification before we get started – I call it "the law of free money". I am more than certain you have heard the many tarnished and occasionally humorous stories of the lottery winners or professional ball players who once had millions of dollars, but are now broke? This is due to the Law of Free Money. If you get something of value without any real effort or expenditure on your part, it really has no value to you, and you eventually lose it. The same goes for your health, weight loss, and whatever other goals you may have. Do you know how many people I see in my practice after a bariatric sur-

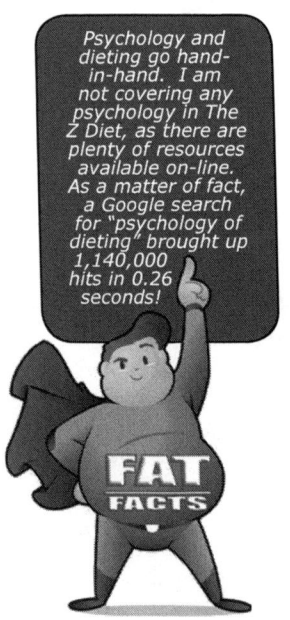

> Psychology and dieting go hand-in-hand. I am not covering any psychology in The Z Diet, as there are plenty of resources available on-line. As a matter of fact, a Google search for "psychology of dieting" brought up 1,140,000 hits in 0.26 seconds!

FAT FACTS

gery has failed them? They underwent severe alteration to their perfectly good, God-given anatomy, without any real effort of their own (especially when insurance or the state pays for it), and they gained all of their weight back and then some. They fought this law, and the law won. Of course there are those who get away with breaking the law, but they are certainly the exception, not the rule. If you want health; if you want to lose weight and maintain the weight loss, it's going to take some effort on your part. Whether it's making time to exercise or preparing your food or thinking ahead before going to a party, you will have to put forth the effort, especially if you are in it for the long term. Make no mistake: if you're after the quick solution, you may be able to obtain it, but chances are you will lose it. The Law of Free Money can't be changed by Congress or overruled by a non-elected federal judge. You will deal with it, unless your solution is full of effort, sweat, and some seriou work. Do not get me wrong – you can do it! Hence the Z Diet. This is a simple solution, but it will still take some effort on your part.

Long term *weight loss maintenance* takes an understanding of a few key principles that I have broken down in the Z Diet. These include, in no particular order of importance:

Understand your starting point

Your starting point is where you are today, and where you will be every day. I consider your starting point something that is continually changing, and that is why I am a big proponent of tracking measurements and/or following some sort of method to see objectively how you are doing. If you think in these terms, that you change your starting point every time you take a measurement or track something, it will remind you to keep it going. The chapter on Body Category Designation is a simplification of that philosophy. I have offered four different *broad* starting points to help direct you in your goal of long term weight loss maintenance. Included in this chapter is some detailed information about insulin, a dieter's best friend and worst enemy. Though this information is listed under the classification The Metabolically Challenged, it is applicable for everyone.

The next chapter covers the Basics of Food, information you must understand in order to maintain long term weight loss. In particular, we will cover the need to keep adequate protein in your eating plan.

The final chapter in the first section is the Z Diet's first look at calories. I use a broad principle called **The Willey Principle** to help you develop an understanding or view of your caloric intake from your current starting point.

Understanding what happens to you when you 'diet'

When you diet, whether for quick weight loss, slow weight loss, or weight loss maintenance, a number of psychological and physiological changes occur. Most of us are quite aware of the obvious ones, so I listed a few that most people, even doctors, do not realize. People's lack of understanding in the areas I've listed is due to the fact that a lot of this information is relatively new and related to a very interesting hormone the fat cell releases, called Leptin. I will not spend a lot of time on Leptin in this book, but I do want you to be aware of what happens to your body and brain as you restrict calories.

I will then follow it with a chapter describing **Quick Weight Loss Approaches.** Why did I include quick weight loss approaches in a long term *weight loss maintenance* book? Once again, I think the information is of great value, not only if you decide to use one of these methods, but to your understanding that real weight loss success is a *lifestyle*, not a diet.

Performance of the Z Diet – Understanding a Lifestyle

The final section of the book is a straightforward breakdown of some key factors in the Z Diet's prescribed lifestyle. These include ways to directly control caloric intake without the tedious job of counting every calorie that crosses your lips. We will also discuss the ways to choose the right amounts of macronutrients (protein, carbohydrates, and fat) for your long term weight loss maintenance plan.

I will then review the Z Diet's incorporation of indirect caloric control, or, more simply put: *how to eat for the rest of your life.* This may be considered the heart of the Z Diet, as I have been using these techniques in my clinical weight loss practice for years, with proven success.

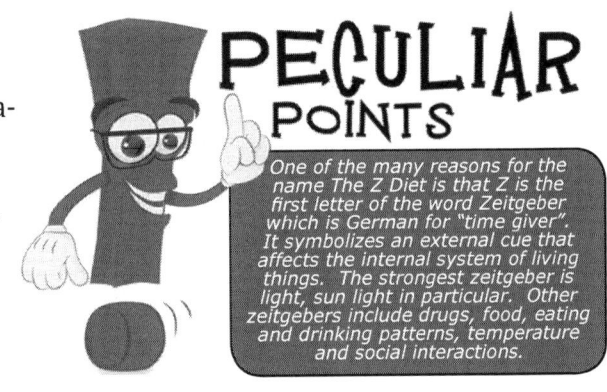

> **PECULIAR POINTS**
>
> One of the many reasons for the name The Z Diet is that Z is the first letter of the word Zeitgeber which is German for "time giver". It symbolizes an external cue that affects the internal system of living things. The strongest zeitgeber is light, sun light in particular. Other zeitgebers include drugs, food, eating and drinking patterns, temperature and social interactions.

Learning How to Shop and Read Labels in the next chapter in the Z Diet, as this too is a component of the lifestyle techniques so vital for your long term success.

Working with your doctor or a board certified Bariatric Physician can be very helpful in your long term weight loss maintenance program, especially important, discussing various medications and their potential role.

Summary

In summary, The Z Diet is about you and *long term weight loss maintenance.* It is a lifestyle, nothing more. Changing your everyday life is not a simple task, but it is very possible. I could provide you incentives, both positive and negative, but it is still up to you to change your life. For whatever reason you picked up this book, know this: The Z Diet works for *long term weight loss maintenance.* I have thousands of people as my witnesses. I would simply encourage you to try. Delve into the information here, take a good hard look at your lifestyle, see where you can work The Z Diet principles in, and go for it!

1. Heymsfield, S.B. et. al. Why do obese patients not lose more weight when treated with low-calorie diets? A mechanistic perspective. Am J Clin Nutr. 2007 Feb;85(2):346-54.

The Z Diet
Your Starting Point

Body Category Designation
Metabolically Challenged
Insulin
Hormonally Challenged
Physique Oriented
General Health

The Basics Of Food

Willey Principle

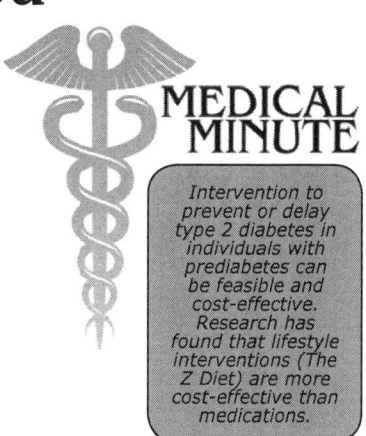

MEDICAL MINUTE

Intervention to prevent or delay type 2 diabetes in individuals with prediabetes can be feasible and cost-effective. Research has found that lifestyle interventions (The Z Diet) are more cost-effective than medications.

2

Body Category Designation

One of the first rules of diet writing is individualization of the eating plans, particularly when it comes to lifelong weight maintenance diet plans. Here is where one of the many difficulties arises when talking to a broad audience – how do I individualize a weight maintenance plan for everyone reading the Z Diet? Well, obviously I can't. What I can do is twofold: 1. I can provide the information and a few key steps in weight loss maintenance, which I hope to accomplish through your reading of this entire book. 2. I can generalize people into one of four categories, based on medical conditions and goals. This will allow me to make suggestions for long term weight loss maintenance and be a little more specific to the individual reading the book. This will obviously not take into account all of the relevant factors in the quest for optimal health and weight loss preservation; however, it will allow some general guidelines for better focus and therefore achievement. I use a similar sorting in my practice as it helps direct people to various programs I offer. The four categories are; *The Metabolically Challenged, The Hormonally Challenged, The Physique Oriented*, and those in quest for *General Health*.

My simple classification method places people with conditions that are responsive to weight loss in any form, but specific attention to macro nutrients, number of calories, etc. may be different for the others. Placing yourself in one of these categories will help you design a long term weight loss maintenance plan that is a little more tailored to you. This simple designation also allows you to go between each one with relative ease. For example, if your goal is physique development, but you are insulin resistant or have diabetes, you can treat your disease state by following the general recommendations of the metabolically challenged eating plan, and then change to the physique oriented plan. Going between the classifications falls right under the benefits of dietary cycling I will be discussing shortly. It also allows me to point out the importance of having your doctor involved with your long term weight loss goals. Your doctor can prescribe hormones and medications, as well as utilize a number of other methodologies to help you with particular classifications you may find yourself in. This chapter will serve to define the conditions, and in the Performing the Z Diet section entitled **Macro Nutrient Breakdown,** I will get into more detail on actual differentiation of long term weight loss eating plans.

The Metabolically Challenged

The most common classification I see in my office is The Metabolically Challenged. The Metabolically Challenged are people who have problems with insulin with or without other medical or hormonal concerns. Simply put, fat or thin, old or young, they have an insulin problem. This could mean they have insulin resistance, diabetes, polycystic ovarian syndrome, or other conditions directly associated with elevated insulin. It goes without saying that insulin and obesity go hand-in-hand: insulin levels rise as the degree of obesity goes up and insulin levels drop with fat loss. I am not going to argue phraseology, I am simply stating that, for the purpose of the Z Diet, if you have a

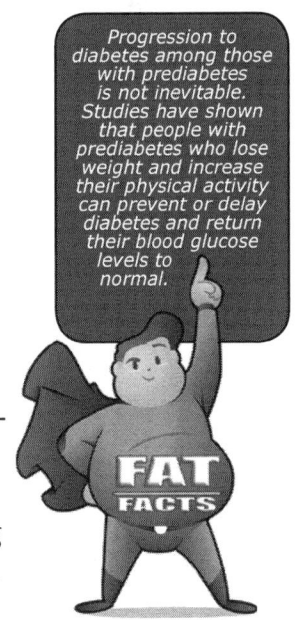

> Progression to diabetes among those with prediabetes is not inevitable. Studies have shown that people with prediabetes who lose weight and increase their physical activity can prevent or delay diabetes and return their blood glucose levels to normal.

FAT FACTS

problem with insulin, you are metabolically challenged. It is simply a way to allow me to direct you toward better lifelong eating habits, based on said problem or concern with insulin. That is it. All other conditions, hormonal issues, and disease states take a back seat when discussing long term weight loss strategies when you are metabolically challenged. I start with this one too, because this is the most predominant condition/classification we see in our weight loss practice. It begs the question of the chicken and the egg; does a problem with insulin cause people to get fat, or does the fat cause a problem with insulin? This is a little beyond the scope of this book, but I think it is vital that everyone know about insulin.

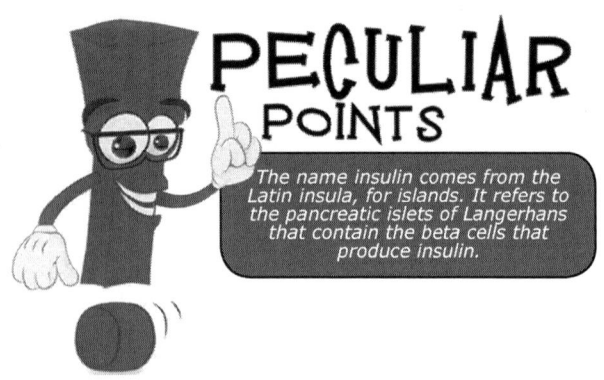

PECULIAR POINTS

The name insulin comes from the Latin insula, for islands. It refers to the pancreatic islets of Langerhans that contain the beta cells that produce insulin.

Insulin

Insulin is likely the mother of all hormones in the discussion of weight loss and lifestyle related disease states. Hormones are powerhouses in the body, responsible for all sorts of different functions, including growth, feelings, etc. Insulin is one of these powerhouses. Insulin is released by the pancreas by a cell called the beta-cell. Insulin, in a normal state, facilitates cellular glucose (sugar) uptake and regulates carbohydrates, fats, and protein metabolism. This hormone is constantly released into the body, but increases in response to nutrients in the blood, and even thoughts of food in the mouth (cephalic phase of insulin release). It responds rapidly according to the type of food consumed, and is influenced most by carbohydrates, followed by protein and fat. The carbohydrates can be broken down further into high glycemic foods and low glycemic foods (see Appendix I – Glycemic Foods). High glycemic foods are absorbed more rapidly, therefore causing a faster release of insulin. Insulin secretion following a meal depends on the amount of the different macronutrients present (is there protein, fat, or fiber present?), the physical form they take (liquid vs. solid), and added or lacking components of the food. Secretion of insulin following a meal also varies according to a number of factors, including how quickly food moves down the track (gastric emptying and motility), gastro-intestinal hormones, and neural input.

One of insulin's actions is to transport sugar in the blood into cells, including muscle, liver, and fat cells. Insulin is not the only hormone that deals with blood sugar. Glucagon, epinephrine (adrenaline) and cortisol also play roles in the fine balancing act of blood sugar control.

So why are we focusing on insulin in our quest for weight loss maintenance and optimal health? Well, for one thing, problems with insulin and blood sugar are a set up for a variety of potentially serious or even life-threatening obstacles, including kidney disease, stroke, eye damage and heart attacks. The zeitgeber sugar, a powerful external force responsible for stimulating Insulin has over-run our society! Estimates run as high as 22 teaspoons of sugar each day, per American! (1,2)

Be sure to note I said *problems* with insulin are dangerous. Insulin in and of itself is wonderful. It is kind of like the gun argument: Guns don't kill people; people kill people and occasionally use guns to do so. Well, insulin does not kill people; people with sugar kill themselves with sugar and insulin is a collaborator! Insulin is a vital hormone. Life is not sustainable without it. Insulin is a powerful muscle building hormone utilized by both performance and physique oriented athletes to increase muscle mass. This is primarily done with food and good eating, but it is also done by taking insulin via a syringe to build muscle (3).

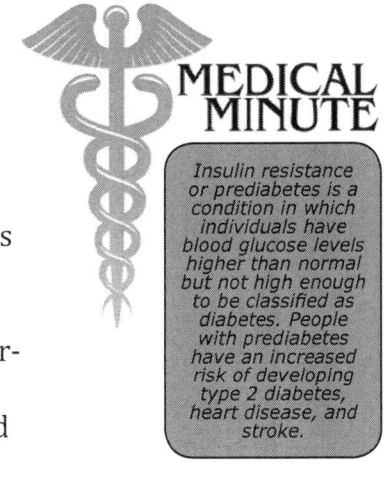

MEDICAL MINUTE

Insulin resistance or prediabetes is a condition in which individuals have blood glucose levels higher than normal but not high enough to be classified as diabetes. People with prediabetes have an increased risk of developing type 2 diabetes, heart disease, and stroke.

The way insulin, and most other hormones for that matter, act is that once stimulated they set up a series of reactions/events throughout the body. It acts by triggering receptors that can be found all over the place on cells throughout the body. Once these receptors 'see' the insulin, it activates specific actions depending on the site the receptor lays.

The term 'insulin sensitivity' simply implies how sensitive the receptor is to the presence of insulin. If the receptors are insulin sensitive, they respond to small amounts of insulin. If they are insulin resistant, a non-derogatory term a few of you may have been called by your doctor, it takes a lot more insulin to pull off the same effects. If the receptors remain insulin resistant for too long, and it takes more and more insulin to achieve the needed effect, you will eventually become diabetic, as the pancreas is no longer able to produce the insulin required to manage all of its essential duties.

Not only is the sensitivity of the insulin receptors important, but also the amount of insulin released once stimulated. There have been theories put into practice, as well as more available research in the area of insulin sensitivity and the actual secretion of insulin after eating. There is an assumption that the factors, insulin receptor sensitivity and amount of insulin released once the pancreas is stimulated, are directly involved with weight gain or loss and the effectiveness of a diet on an individual. This is important, as determining what your insulin sensitivity is, as well as how you secrete insulin, may be essential in long term weight loss. This is also very hard to do. There are a few protocols that combine the phlebotomist's needle and a doctor's prescription; however, it is even harder to interpret the results. This is beyond the scope of The Z Diet. If you are interested, a simpler and, in my opinion, just as effective way to determine how the zeitgeber food affects you and your insulin, is to attempt different styles of eating plans. This would involve alternating low carb dieting with high carb dieting and keeping track of how your body changes, how you feel, etc. I have outlined this in more detail in one of my earlier books, **Better Than Steroids**.

I have developed a simple questionnaire to help you determine whether you are insulin sensitive, insulin resistant, a high insulin secretor, or a low/normal insulin secretor. This, admittedly, is not science at its finest. This is a simple questionnaire I use in clinical practice to help me establish two things: 1. Does this patient need more testing? 2. What macronutrient content of his or her eating plan should I start him or her on (amount of carbohydrates, proteins, and fat)?

Insulin Sensitivity Questionnaire

This is a simple "test" to help you determine if you may be insulin resistant. Answer the questions on a 5 point scale, 1 being strongly disagree and 5 being strongly agree. Once complete, add your scores to help you determine if you have an insulin problem.

1. **My fat distribution is around my belly (i.e. my arms and legs are not where I hold fat).**

Strongly Disagree	Disagree	Neutral	Agree	Strongly Agree
1	2	3	4	5

2. **I have a hard time losing weight, no matter how hard I exercise or diet.**

Strongly Disagree	Disagree	Neutral	Agree	Strongly Agree
1	2	3	4	5

3. **I feel extremely drained after lunch and want to take a nap.**

Strongly Disagree	Disagree	Neutral	Agree	Strongly Agree
1	2	3	4	5

4. **After eating a meal in which the majority is carbohydrates (breads, pasta, cereal, sweets, etc.), I feel full, dumpy and rather bloated.**

Strongly Disagree	Disagree	Neutral	Agree	Strongly Agree
1	2	3	4	5

5. **After eating a meal in which the majority is carbohydrates (breads, pasta, cereal, sweets, etc.) I get an energy crash, fall asleep easily, and find myself hungry and looking for more food.**

Strongly Disagree	Disagree	Neutral	Agree	Strongly Agree
1	2	3	4	5

TOTAL: _____

If you scored between 21 and 25, more than likely you are insulin resistant. You may want to visit with your primary care provider to confirm this with a medical consult and possibly some blood tests. Your solution should also consist of following The Z Diet to a tee.

If you scored between 15 and 20, you are border-lining a problem. You most certainly need to follow The Z Diet as best you can. You may want to consider seeing your doctor as well before it progresses to a problem.

If you scored between 11 and 14, you are in a grey zone (there is always a grey zone…) and it could be part of the reason you are not dropping the fat like you may have in the past. You can likely reverse any problems you have simply by following the solutions provided in The Z Diet.

If you scored less than 10, congratulations! Use the Z Diet to perfect your eating habits and health, and possibly even zero in on that physique you want! Many professional athletes as well as people in extremely good shape score in this area. They are more likely to answer the questions with a 1 or 2, and in response to question number 4, they tell me they feel tremendously energized by a carbohydrate meal. The weight lifters and bodybuilders tell me they get a literal 'pump' in all of their muscles when eating carbohydrates, as if they have just left the gym. One of their secrets may be the ability to optimize that powerful hormone called insulin.

No matter how you scored, if you answered 4 or 5 to question number 5, you are likely an insulin hyper-secretor. In other words, you produce too much insulin. There are a number of potential causes, including the fact that you need more insulin to get the same amount of work done (i.e. insulin resistance). This can be modifiable with the suggestions listed below, including supplements. There are even some drugs your doctor can prescribe to benefit you in this area.

MEDICAL MINUTE

In 2003–2006, 25.9% of U.S. adults age 20 years or older had IFG (35.4% of adults aged 60 years or older). Applying this percentage to the entire U.S. population in 2007 yields an estimated 57 million American adults age 20 years or older with IFG, suggesting that at least 57 million American adults had prediabetes in 2007.

No matter what your baseline insulin response is, or how functional or dysfunctional your insulin receptors are, increasing insulin sensitivity is something the Z Diet does and its applications can be applied across the board. Incorporating even one application of The Z Diet will increase insulin sensitivity; however, like many things in life, the more the better!

Let's cover a few more important facts about insulin that will help you understand its role in weight loss. The actions of insulin are immense and numerous. I am going to discuss a few of insulin's primary actions as they relate to long term weight loss.

Insulin Increases Protein Synthesis

Insulin increases transport of amino acids into muscle cells, which is essential in building and maintaining lean muscle mass. Insulin has been called the most anabolic or growth promoting hormone in the body. Fine tuning of eating and even using insulin from a syringe (3) are very powerful mechanisms utilized by some to build muscle mass. In the non-athletic world, lean mass is essential not only in all aspects of health and disease prevention, but is also directly correlated with that elusive metabolism everyone claims has left them!

Insulin Decreases the Breakdown of Protein (proteolysis)

Insulin reduces protein degradation (break down) by inhibiting the use of amino acids, the building block of protein, for making sugar for the body to use as energy. This process is called gluconeogenesis, or the production of sugar from non-sugar basics and it occurs in the liver. This is important not only because of the role of muscle mass in metabolic processes and disease state management/prevention, but also in some of the pathopysiology of diabetes.

Insulin Antagonizes Cortisol

Cortisol is essential for life itself. It is often called the stress hormone, as it responds to stress and anxiety in a protective way by raising blood pressure and blood sugar. However, as you are likely aware from all of the info-commercials about 'anti-cortisol' supplements, it is considered one of the bad guys in the battle of the belly. High cortisol levels have been linked with decreased insulin sensitivity in muscles and liver and increased insulin sensitivity in fat tissue. (4-6). Cortisol is also a direct antagonist of insulin by increasing gluconeogenesis and the breakdown of proteins.

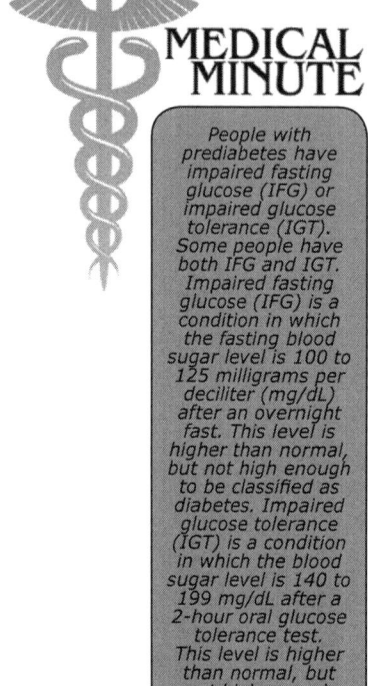

Insulin Inhibits Lipolysis

This is of prime importance, especially in the weight/fat loss arena. When insulin is elevated, particularly after a high glycemic meal, your body cannot, will not, under any circumstance, burn fat or use fat for energy. It is a very protective mechanism, best described by this analogy: When our great-great-great grandfathers all where hunting and gathering across the lands of their time, they had periods of great eating, and periods of great hunger. As a protective mechanism, the body – when food was present and therefore insulin was elevated – would focus on storage of nutrients. Insulin would inhibit the use of fat as plenty of food was available via the mouth. During times of hunger, insulin secretion would decrease and the body was allowed access to fat stores for energy. This same mechanism is still at play today even though we rarely (thankfully...) go hungry. Maybe part of our obesity problem? You bet it is!

MEDICAL MINUTE

People with prediabetes have impaired fasting glucose (IFG) or impaired glucose tolerance (IGT). Some people have both IFG and IGT. Impaired fasting glucose (IFG) is a condition in which the fasting blood sugar level is 100 to 125 milligrams per deciliter (mg/dL) after an overnight fast. This level is higher than normal, but not high enough to be classified as diabetes. Impaired glucose tolerance (IGT) is a condition in which the blood sugar level is 140 to 199 mg/dL after a 2-hour oral glucose tolerance test. This level is higher than normal, but not high enough to be classified as diabetes.

As I mentioned previously, insulin responds most quickly to high glycemic foods like sugar, followed by other types of carbohydrates and proteins based on a number of factors. If insulin is continually elevated, due to your diet, your sensitivity lessens, secretion increases to try to combat the increasing resistance and you are officially in the fatness cycle. High insulin secretion then causes you to be hungry and your vicious cycle just went downhill.

As I mentioned above, insulin prevents lipolysis or the breakdown of fat, so you gain more fat, increasing insulin resistance, increasing insulin secretion and now that cycle has come to a cliff, and you're not stopping it from rolling...

So how do we break this vicious cycle? First and foremost, lose weight! Then control your insulin by following the suggestions of the Z Diet. Second, via the Z Diet and the information given below, increase insulin sensitivity, and third, start burning fat instead of storing it, thereby decreasing the amount of insulin resistance and insulin release. Can you see the positive/ beneficial cycle starting?

There are a number of mechanisms by which insulin inhibits the breakdown of fat. They are somewhat tedious and therefore will not be provided in great detail. It is important to say, however, that a number of everyday activities will allow an increase in insulin sensitivity and a decrease in insulin secretion, thereby creating the environment for fat burning.

Increasing Insulin Sensitivity

The following lists are additional ways to increase your insulin sensitivity, thereby increasing your fat loss:

In the big picture: Avoid certain foods

I tell people all the time that there is no such thing as a bad food, just bad diets. In saying this I avoid criminalizing foods, but it also allows me to offer a solution to those foods. That solution is simple. The majority of time, avoid foods that are high in sugar, refined, processed, and liquid. In particular, since this section is about insulin, avoid the high sugar, and refined, processed, and liquid carbohydrates! A number of people refer to these types of foods as high glycemic or impact carbs. I call them active carbohydrates. I will cover them in a little more detail in The Basics of Food and Appendix I – Glycemic Foods.

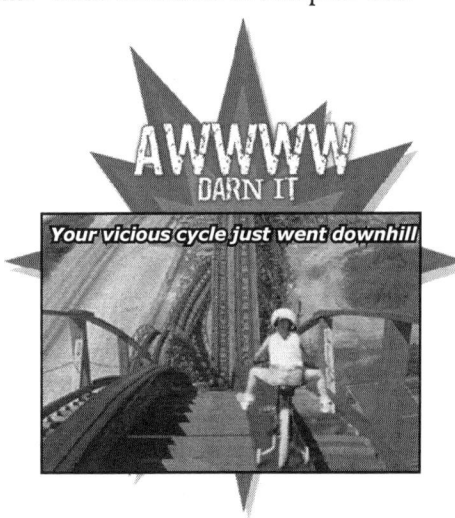

When you eat carbohydrates think: *PFFV*!

PFFV stands for ***P**rotein, **F**at, **F**iber* and ***V**egetables*. Any or all of these added to a carbohydrate burdened meal will slow the insulin response, via a few different mechanisms. In general, all of them will decrease the rate of absorption of the carbohydrate, thereby slowing insulin's response. Protein also has the additive effect of stimulating the release of glucagon. This antagonizes insulin directly. Fiber can really slow down the rate at which sugar hits the blood stream, thereby causing insulin to respond more slowly as well. Adding a fiber supplement such as glucomannan, inulin, or psyllium husk is a simple way to do that. Vegetables add vitamins, minerals, and fiber to your meal and also help to change the insulin response. And, like your mom told you, they are good for you!

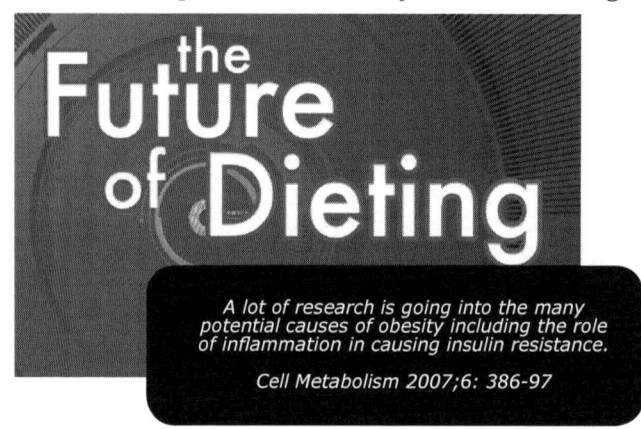

The Future of Dieting

A lot of research is going into the many potential causes of obesity including the role of inflammation in causing insulin resistance.

Cell Metabolism 2007;6: 386-97

Exercise

The effects of exercise are profound to say the least. So powerful are the effects that one exercise session, in someone with insulin resistance, will increase their insulin sensitivity (7,8). One session! And it is already working. Exercise also increases long term insulin sensitivity. Though exercise will not directly cause changes in your weight, what a simple solution to the primary problem of insulin sensitivity.

Supplements

A few over-the-counter supplements are also of great benefit to increasing insulin sensitivity. Omega-3 Fatty Acids top my list for increasing insulin sensitivity via supplements (9,10), with fish oil being the best way to get it. It takes a good dose (10-12 grams/day) and you need to be sure to find a good reputable brand with the proper ratio of DHA/EPA. Alpha-Lipoic-Acid is of benefit as a powerful antioxidant as well as a modifier of insulin sensitivity. A dose of 100 to 200 mg per carb filled meal is adequate. Low levels of dietary Magnesium have been associated with insulin resistance (11-13). I suggest having your levels checked by your doctor if you are insulin resistant and/or start taking 500 mg/day and slowly increase from there. If you take too much too fast, you will benefit your insulin resistance by increasing your exercise - by running to the bathroom...Remember when mom gave you Milk-of-magnesia when you where a little backed up as a kid? The active ingredient is magnesium.

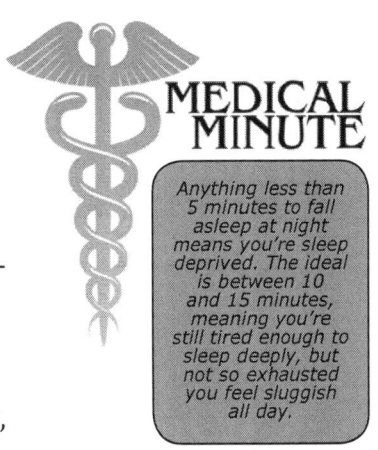

> **MEDICAL MINUTE**
> Anything less than 5 minutes to fall asleep at night means you're sleep deprived. The ideal is between 10 and 15 minutes, meaning you're still tired enough to sleep deeply, but not so exhausted you feel sluggish all day.

Zinc is another supplement that could potentially help with insulin resistance. Zinc is important in insulin biosynthesis and secretion and is concentrated in the pancreas. Chromium deficiency has been associated with glucose intolerance and insulin resistance in patients on long term IV nutrition, and may be of some benefit in insulin resistance.

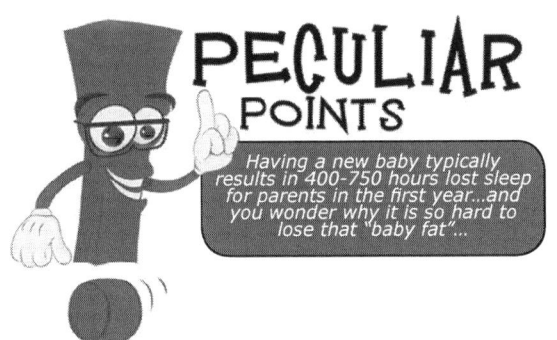

> **PECULIAR POINTS**
> Having a new baby typically results in 400-750 hours lost sleep for parents in the first year...and you wonder why it is so hard to lose that "baby fat"...

Sleep

No sleep – no weight loss. This is backed by studies that indicate the same. Sleep deprivation raises fasting blood sugars and alters cortisol production in healthy young adults (14). There is also plenty of evidence that chronic sleep deprivation impacts insulin and insulin resistance and increases weight (15). Sleep deprivation is associated with decreased concentrations of leptin (a hormone produced by fat that regulates fat mass and appetite) and increases in ghrelin, a gut hormone that increases appetite (16). Obstructive sleep apnea, a condition where sleep is disrupted due to inadequate oxygen, causes impaired sugar tolerance independent of obesity (17). Solution?

Get your sleep! If you have difficulty sleeping (true insomnia), visit with your doctor for some elucidation. If you have alternating shifts at work that mess with your sleep cycle, The Z Diet and utilizing low dose, over-the-counter melatonin will help.

After providing this information I am asked all the time by my patients: "Can I get off my diabetes medicines if I adhere to The Z Diet, exercise every day, and take my supplements as you suggest?" That is very difficult to answer in a one-on-one setting, and nearly impossible in a book. The variables involved are tremendous, and far too tedious for our discussion. Let me say this: I would never discourage anyone by telling them they can never come off their medications if they adhere to a good eating and exercise program. I would encourage you to talk to your doctor about your eating and exercise program, and as you make headway, discuss alterations in your medication regimen – something we will cover shortly.

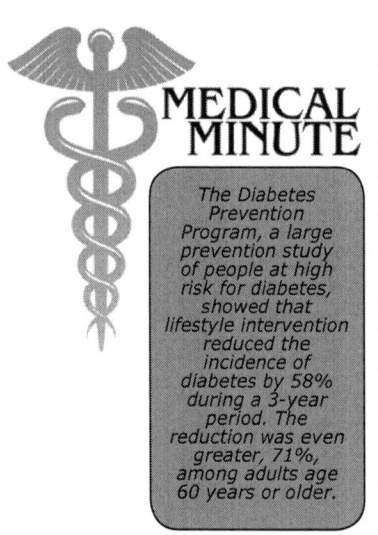

MEDICAL MINUTE

The Diabetes Prevention Program, a large prevention study of people at high risk for diabetes, showed that lifestyle intervention reduced the incidence of diabetes by 58% during a 3-year period. The reduction was even greater, 71%, among adults age 60 years or older.

I am hopeful that you now understand the implications, importance, consequences and solutions for that wonderful, yet potentially devastating hormone, insulin. I want to leave you with one more thought before we move on. One would think that the primary reason I am consulted in my weight loss practice is weight loss. It's not. The number one reason people seek my advice is to help them combat fatigue. They are keenly aware that their weight has a lot to do with that chief complaint, but all else considered, fatigue and an inability to function at their desired capacity are the top reasons people see me. Why do I mention this in the chapter on insulin?

Time for medical school 101: Histology. Histology is a branch of anatomy concerned with the study of the microscopic structures of animal and plant tissue. One of the microscopic organs we focus on in everything from disease states to professional sports is called mitochondria. Mitochondria are sometimes described as the power houses of the cell because they generate most of the cell's supply of energy, adenosine triphosphate (ATP) to be exact. In addition to supplying cellular energy, mitochondria are involved in a range of other processes, such as signaling, cellular differentiation, and cell death, as well as the control of the cell cycle and cell growth (14). They may also be directly involved in the aging process itself! Continually elevated insulin levels as seen in insulin resistance and elevated insulin secretion have been shown to damage and prevent the creation of new mitochondria. In other words, there may be a very good reason and a simple intervention for your fatigue. Follow The Z Diet, lower your insulin levels, increase your insulin sensitivity and guess what? More energy!!

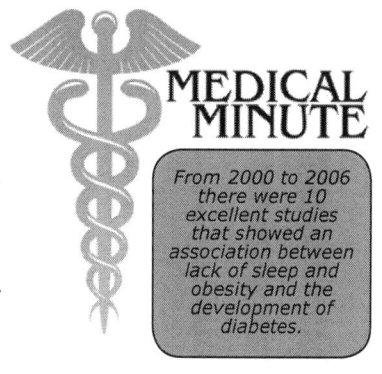

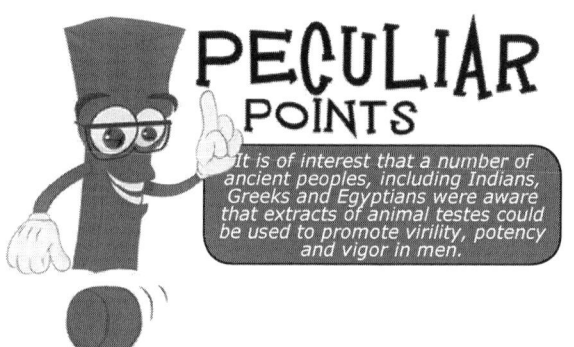

MEDICAL MINUTE
From 2000 to 2006 there were 10 excellent studies that showed an association between lack of sleep and obesity and the development of diabetes.

PECULIAR POINTS
It is of interest that a number of ancient peoples, including Indians, Greeks and Egyptians were aware that extracts of animal testes could be used to promote virility, potency and vigor in men.

In the performance section of the Z Diet I will be discussing a theme I call Food Timing, an essential aspect of The Z Diet. The Z Diet in general and Food Timing in particular work hand-in-hand with insulin to get all of the good benefits from the hormone, and help negate the bad things insulin can do. I will be referring to insulin a lot and even be demonstrating food timing using insulin as our model.

The Hormonally Challenged

The Hormonally Challenged individual is a male or female with *non-pancreatic related hormone problems*. Recall from above, if you have insulin problems, they override all other categories as described in The Z Diet, so if you fall under the hormonally challenged, your insulin is 'fine', but any of the other hormones in the body are wreaking havoc. In general, these would be problems with the sex hormones such as testosterone, estrogen, and progesterone, or problems with your thyroid, adrenal glands, and the pituitary hormone/protein, Human Growth Hormone (hGH). Specifically, and speaking strictly in terms

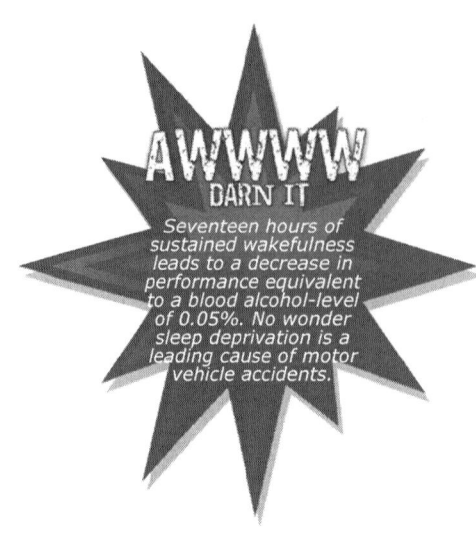

> **AWWWW DARN IT**
> Seventeen hours of sustained wakefulness leads to a decrease in performance equivalent to a blood alcohol-level of 0.05%. No wonder sleep deprivation is a leading cause of motor vehicle accidents.

of the sex hormones, in the female this could be peri-menopause or menopause and may even be considered post-menopause by some. In the male, and once again speaking specifically about the sex hormones, it would be testosterone deficiency or Andropause. I am not going to cover these problems per say in the Z Diet book. You can find more information about them in my book ***What Does Your Doctor Look Like Naked? Your Guide to Optimal Health***.

Obviously, this is one area your doctor may be able to help you with. I am also classifying individuals into this category because if you feel you have a problem with your hormones, it behooves you to talk with your health care provider about them. It is most certainly of great benefit to have well balanced, well regulated, optimized hormones in your pursuit of long term weight loss maintenance. Specific eating regimens and supplements help with hormonal balance as well. Without going into a lot of detail here, my favorite supplement for proper hormone balance is Diindolyl Methane or DIM, at a dose of 200 to 400 mg once or twice a day. There are a number of other supplements that help with both male and female hormone balance and optimization, but again, that is not the purpose of this book.

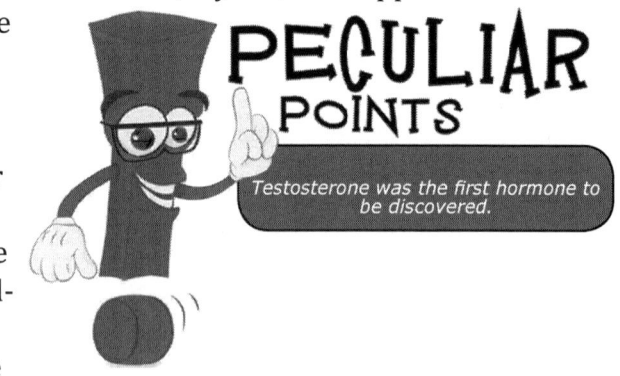

> **PECULIAR POINTS**
> Testosterone was the first hormone to be discovered.

The Physique Oriented

The Physique Oriented person is someone of average risk, without medical problems or concerns, whose primary goal is physique development. This means they do not have metabolic or hormonal concerns, as defined above, when they set out for their long term maintenance plan. If you are larger when you start this approach (percent body fat greater than 25 for a male and 30 for a female), check with your doctor for some lab work and an evaluation to be sure you do not fall into the metabolically challenged category. You could also take the Insulin Questionnaire for a little direction.

The Physique Oriented person differs in a few key areas in long term weight loss maintenance in the sense that vigorous exercise must be a part of his or her daily regimen. Exercise plans are beyond the scope of this book, but I have a number of sample plans available for download on my website www.eatright4u.com.

General Health

This is the classification for the person who has recently lost weight and wants to maintain it for life, who is not metabolically challenged, does not have hormonal issues, and does not have a lot of physique goals other than never gaining his or her weight back. In my experience, this could apply to anyone who has found successful weight loss, but who now needs a way to keep it off.

In concluding this chapter, my goal is simply to allow more individualization of your long term eating plans and, as was likely obvious, to preach a little about insulin. I will be referring to each of these categories throughout the book. The Performance of the Z Diet itself is your best bet for long term weight loss success, with or without ever classifying yourself into one of these four categories. They are simply offered as a guide to provide a little more individuality to the suggestions outlined.

1. American Heart Association, http://www.americanheart.org/nutrition/sugar

2. U.S. Department of Agriculture's database listing added sugars in certain foods, http://tinyurl.com/nacqhr

3. The Physician and Sports Medicine. INSULIN AS AN ANABOLIC AID?: A DANGER FOR STRENGTH ATHLETES. by: J. Warren Willey II, DO *Volume: 25, Issue: 10, Published: October 1997, Clinical Article*

4. Reinehr, T and Andler W. Cortisol and its relation to insulin resistance before and after weight loss in obese children. *Horm Res.* 2004;62(3):107-12. Epub 2004 Jul 15.

5. De Luca C and Olefsky JM. Stressed out about obesity and insulin resistance. *Nat Med.* 2006 Jan;12(1):41-2

6. Andrews RC and Walker BR. Glucocorticoids and insulin resistance: old hormones, new targets. *Clin Sci (Lond).* 1999 May;96(5):513-23. Review.

7. Ren JM et al. Exercise induces rapid increases in GLUT4 expression, glucose transport capacity, and insulin-stimulated glycogen storage in muscle. *J Biol Chem.* 1994 May 20;269(20):14396-401.

8. Smutok MA, Reece C, Kokkinos PF, et al. Effects of exercise training modality on glucose tolerance in men with abnormal glucose regulation. *Int J Sports Med* 1994;15:283-9.

9. Popp-Snijders C. Dietary supplementation of omega-3 polyunsaturated fatty acids improves insulin sensitivity in non-insulin-dependent diabetes. *Diabetes Res.* 1987 Mar;4(3):141-7.

10. Lovejoy, JC. The influence of dietary fat on insulin resistance. *Current Diabetes Reports.* 2002 2 (5): 435-440.

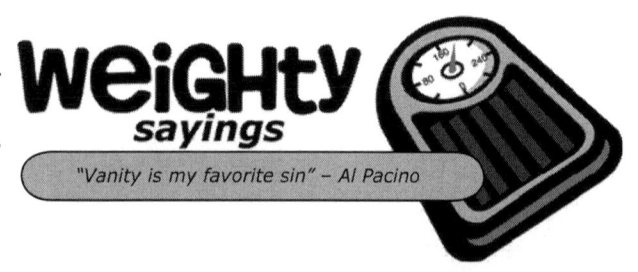

WeiGHty sayings

"Vanity is my favorite sin" – Al Pacino

11. Humphries S, Kushner H, Falkner B. Low dietary magnesium is associated with insulin resistance in a sample of young, nondiabetic Black Americans. *Am J Hypertens* 1999;12:747-56.

12. Rosolova H, Mayer O Jr, Reaven G. Effect of variations in plasma magnesium concentration on resistance to insulin-mediated glucose disposal in nondiabetic subjects. *J Clin Endocrinol Metab* 1997;82:3783-5.

13. Nadler JL, Buchanan T, Natarajan R, et al. Magnesium deficiency produces insulin resistance and increased thromboxane synthesis. *Hypertension* 1993;21:1024-9.

14. Spiegel K, Leproult R, Van Cauter E. Impact of sleep debt on metabolic and endocrine function. Lancet. 1999;354:1435–9.

15. Vorona RD, Winn MP, Babineau TW, Eng BP, Feldman HR, Ware JC. Overweight and obese patients in a primary care population report less sleep than patients with a normal body mass index. Arch Intern Med. 2005;165:25–30

16. Spiegel K, Tasali E, Penev P, Van Cauter E. Sleep curtailment in healthy young men is associated with decreased leptin levels, elevated ghrelin levels, and increased hunger and appetite. Ann Intern Med. 2004;141:846–50.

17. Tassone F, Lanfranco F, Gianotti L, et al. Obstructive sleep apnoea syndrome impairs insulin sensitivity independently of anthropometric variables. Clin Endocrinol (Oxf). 2003;59:374–9.

18. McBride HM, Neuspiel M, Wasiak S (2006). "Mitochondria: more than just a powerhouse". *Curr. Biol.* **16** (14): R551.

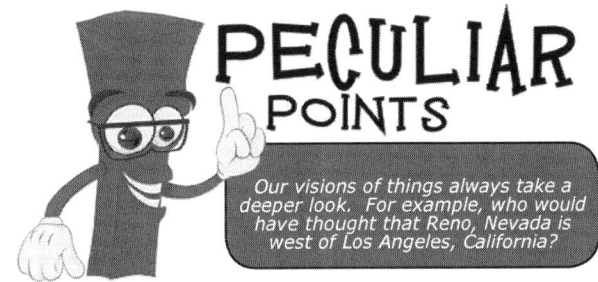

PECULIAR POINTS

Our visions of things always take a deeper look. For example, who would have thought that Reno, Nevada is west of Los Angeles, California?

3

The Basics Of Food

Every one of my books contains the following information about food. I am amazed and occasionally stumped by the fact that so many of the people I see do not know what a carbohydrate is, or what a protein does, etc. To many, this will be a review, and we all need it! To the rest, in relation to The Z Diet this is your Pharmacology 101 class. Food is a drug. This information is vital to your success. This chapter will be reviewing nutrients in the diet. I will review calories in much more detail in coming chapters and just make a brief statement about the caloric content of the nutrients under their respective headings.

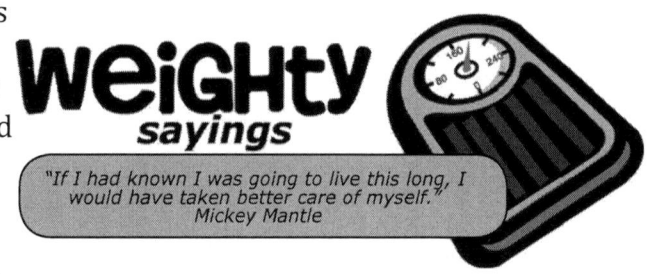

weiGHty sayings

"If I had known I was going to live this long, I would have taken better care of myself."
Mickey Mantle

Essential, Semi-Essential, and Non-Essential Nutrients

It is very important that I clarify essential vs. non-essential foods and semi-essential foods. Understanding this is part of a long term weight management program. Essential foods are foods your body cannot produce on its own, but which are absolutely needed for survival. Examples include, in general, proteins and, more specifically, certain amino acids found in proteins. A few of the fatty acids are in this group as well. Semi-essential foods may be needed under certain conditions/circumstances. Examples of these foods include certain 'non-essential' amino acids (meaning these amino acids can be synthesized by the body using other amino acids) such as L – Glutamine that becomes essential due to heavy exercise. Carbohydrates fall into this category. Non-essential foods are foods that the body can survive without. In non-exercising, non-active individuals, with or without metabolic challenges, carbohydrates meet this requirement. I always get a kick out of the fact that the diet gurus who work for the government admit that carbohydrates are non-essential, but then suggest that all of our diets, no matter what you do or what medical problems you may have, consist of 55+ percent carbohydrates!

The reason this is important for long term weight maintenance is to help you understand one of the basic concepts of the Z Diet. Essential nutrients must be a regular and consistent part of your diet. Semi-essential nutrients should be utilized when they are needed, for example, carbohydrates, including active ones, if you participate in heavy exercise or sports. Non-essential nutrients do not have to be avoided, just controlled. I will cover this in much more detail as we continue in to the fundamentals of The Z Diet.

Carbohydrates

Contrary to the message of some popular diet plans, carbohydrates are *not* bad. Remember, there is no such thing as a bad food, only bad choices, bad timing and bad diets! Carbohydrates contain approximately 4 calories per gram. So if you eat 10 grams of a simple carbohydrate, you get 40 calories from it. Carbohydrates, in particular the active ones, may not be optimal for some people (based on medical conditions i.e. the metabolically challenged and/or genetics) but they are certainly not bad. Carbohydrates are essential for energy, especially the energy needed for sports, exercise, and building muscles! They play a vital role in the body's ability to increase lean mass, and fuel the body. A few body tissues rely solely on glucose for energy including the brain (however the brain can use fatty acids indirectly – a topic out of context for this book), a portion of the kidney called the renal medulla, red blood cells, white blood cells, and peripheral nerves. The body is simply amazing when it comes to utilizing energy sources. When carbohydrates/sugars are available, your body uses them. When they are not, other energy sources such as fat and proteins are utilized. For purposes of The Z Diet we will define carbohydrates as two primary types: **Active and Free**

Active Carbohydrates are also called, depending on whose terminology you prefer, starchy carbohydrates, white carbohydrates, high glycemic carbohydrates, and impact carbs. These drugs have a powerful affect on the hormonal and biochemical systems of the body; hence *active carbohydrates*. Now it goes without saying that all foods have some influence; however, and again for our purposes, we are looking at food in the big picture as it relates to your optimum health and weight loss maintenance. Active carbohydrates cause a rise in blood sugar, the rate dependant on the glycemic index of the food (continue reading and see Appendix I), and a resulting rise in insulin, the hormone responsible for getting sugar out of the blood and into tissues, including muscles and fat. I consider these active because they have a direct influence on your energy, thought processes, cravings, emotions, and body in terms of lean and fat mass. These carbohydrates, as I stated earlier, are not bad, nor should they be avoided. They just need to be regulated, particularly in people who are metabolically challenged. As a matter of fact, when used correctly these nutrients are very powerful and can be essential in helping you reach any fitness or body goal you may have. What do I mean by correctly? How can carbohydrates be utilized in weight loss maintenance?

One of my main focuses in life and dieting is building and maintaining lean mass (read any of my books or articles). Carbohydrates are needed, to some degree, to prevent lean mass break-down over time. This is one of the primary reasons I talk about no carb diets (ketogentic diets or Keto Runs) being short term for most people. Carbohydrates stimulate insulin, which antagonizes cortisol (a hormone whose job description includes making sugar out of muscle to feed the body). Eating carbs also feeds your brain so it does not order biceps for breakfast.

This brings up the next question I get hit with in clinical practice all the time: "So doc, how many carbohydrates should I have in a day?" This question can potentially be answered if you are sitting in my office because I will know you, your goals, your medical condition, your emotional condition, your cravings, your roadblocks, etc. In other words, your goals, needs, how well you function with or without carbohydrates, whether you are metabolically challenged, all play a role in answering that question. Carbohydrates are non-essential nutrients. The only way I can answer that in a book is to say, "The more active you are, the more active carbohydrates you need." The requirements of a tri-athlete are far greater than those of a desk jockey. The desk jockey's requirements will change if he or she decides to take up a regular exercise program. That is as specific as I can get in this setting. If you were to come to my office, fill out a load of paper work, and let me visit with you, I could answer that question more precisely.

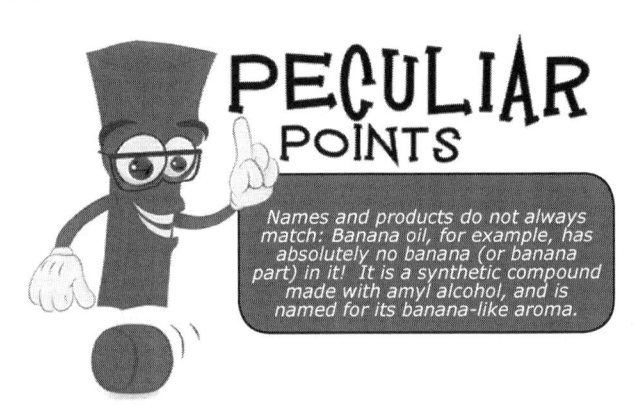

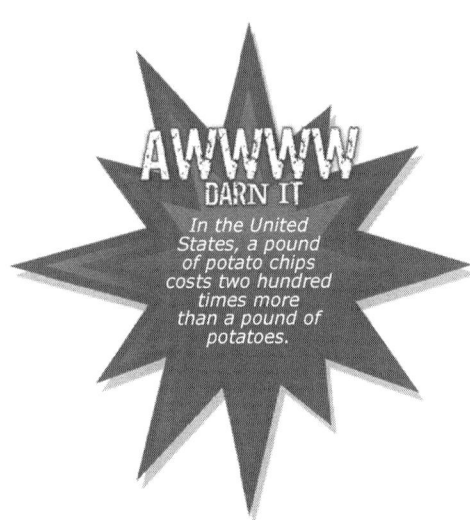

PECULIAR POINTS

Names and products do not always match: Banana oil, for example, has absolutely no banana (or banana part) in it! It is a synthetic compound made with amyl alcohol, and is named for its banana-like aroma.

AWWWW DARN IT

In the United States, a pound of potato chips costs two hundred times more than a pound of potatoes.

This is an excerpt from two of my other books, but it has served me well in all the years I have been teaching weight loss to my clients. It provides a simple visual for judging amounts of this non-essential nutrient, particularly in people that are after fat loss: Get a cup, and place it right in front of you. Imagine that cup as your ability to handle active carbohydrates. When that cup is half full, your body will utilize the energy from the carbohydrates and the energy from fat. As that cup approaches 'fullness', however, the body is more inclined to utilize the energy from the active carbohydrates, and leave the fat alone (survivalist response). When you eat too many active carbohydrates, or you eat them at the wrong time of day, 'the cup runneth over' and that excess is stored as fat! At the opposite extreme, when that cup is empty, your body has little energy to perform activities of daily living and exercise.

This analogy is also applicable to utilizing the prescribed dietary break or the free window (covered in detail in the performance section of the Z Diet). Though not essential all the time, one method of using the free window is to purposely drain the cup by eating a lower active carbohydrate plan for a few days prior to your free window, and filling the cup up with your free window.

Free Carbohydrates

Free carbohydrates are also called fibrous carbohydrates, non-active carbohydrates, low glycemic carbohydrates, and non-impact carbs. These are the carbohydrates that do not have the dramatic affect on blood sugar and insulin that active carbohydrates do. They are weaker drugs unless their external force causes some internal bowel activity.

Free carbohydrates can be utilized whenever and as often as you need them. They are great fillers, adding bulk to your diet, as well as satisfying that strong oral fixation we all have. They are water and air filled, and full of fiber and (except for a few of them) vitamin packed. They provide a variety of tastes and textures that we need when following an eating program. Simply put, they are good for you!

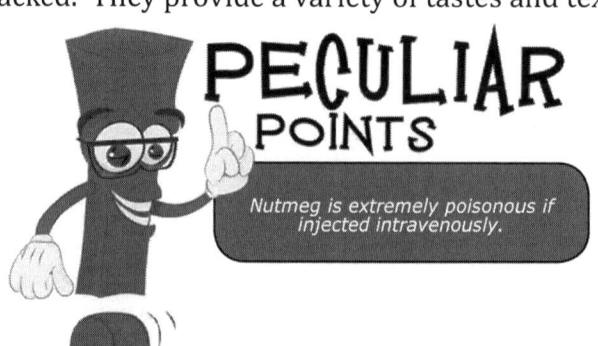

FAT FACTS: Potatoes are not bad (yes I live in Idaho...) – they are packed to the hilt with nutrients! As a matter of fact, the only essential vitamin not found in the white potato is Vitamin A.

PECULIAR POINTS

Nutmeg is extremely poisonous if injected intravenously.

Proteins

The word protein is derived from the Greek word meaning **of prime importance**.

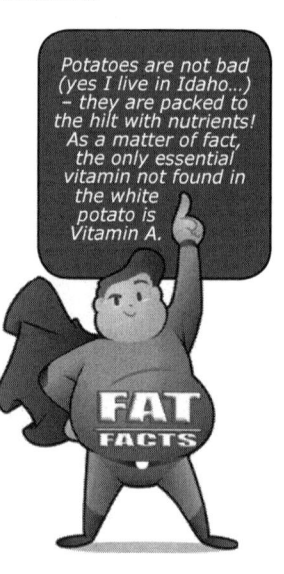

try's nutrition advisors, has been said can cause kidney damage, as a simple error in logic dictated that those with kidney damage need to decrease the amount of protein they take in (1). To my knowledge, there has never been a study showing that people with normal kidney function will damage their kidneys with high intakes of protein. It is an unfortunate myth, as without question in my clinical practice (before people get to me) their protein intake is too low.

High protein intake also gets unfairly blamed for poor bone health. I have never met anyone, particularly athletes, who takes a lot of protein and has poor bones, but my observation really means little. The concern is that high protein intake changes the bone-calcium interaction. It is far more complex than I care to get into here, but suffice it to say that when your calcium and vitamin D intake are appropriate, protein plays a vital role in preserving bone health (2). In situations of high protein intake in the presence of low calcium and vitamin D intake, there may be potential harm. Simple solution? Take your calcium and vitamin D as your doctor always recommends.

High protein intake in the form of meat has had many a crooked finger pointed at it over concerns of cancer and heart disease. Recently, I have seen a number of studies contradicting this. Why the confusion? I think it has to do more with the fact that a lot of modern meats are processed and the more popular ones have a large amount of fat, in particular saturated fat. High fat intake in America has been associated with low intake of fruits and vegetables, known protectors of the body from cancer and heart disease. Simply put: there are a number of factors involved in both cancer and heart disease, and placing all the blame on a high protein based diet, without including other

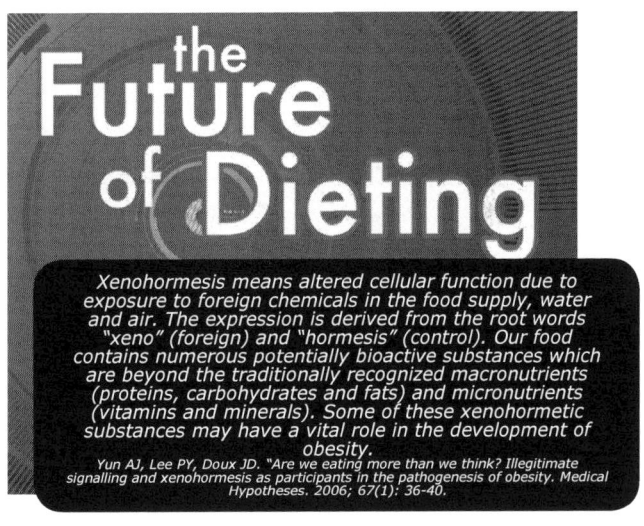

> **the Future of Dieting**
>
> Xenohormesis means altered cellular function due to exposure to foreign chemicals in the food supply, water and air. The expression is derived from the root words "xeno" (foreign) and "hormesis" (control). Our food contains numerous potentially bioactive substances which are beyond the traditionally recognized macronutrients (proteins, carbohydrates and fats) and micronutrients (vitamins and minerals). Some of these xenohormetic substances may have a vital role in the development of obesity.
> Yun AJ, Lee PY, Doux JD. "Are we eating more than we think? Illegitimate signalling and xenohormesis as participants in the pathogenesis of obesity. Medical Hypotheses. 2006; 67(1): 36-40.

MEDICAL MINUTE

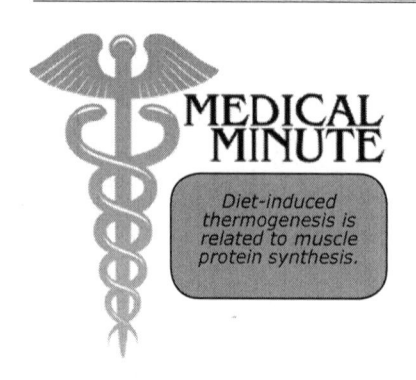

Diet-induced thermogenesis is related to muscle protein synthesis.

variables, is unfortunate.

Now that I have, I hope, put to rest some common myths of high protein diets, it begs the question how much protein do you need? We have established that protein is an essential nutrient. I am also one-hundred percent convinced that adequate protein must be consumed on a regular basis for you to be successful with long term weight loss. Addressing this question involves some difficulty, but it is a little easier than the "how many carbohydrates do I need?" The RDA recommends that 0.8 g/kg or 0.36 g/lb is sufficient protein for everyone, no matter what their goal is, activity level is, starting point is, etc. Obviously, I am about to disagree with that. Protein requirements for athletes, particularly strength and power athletes, far exceeds this, but this is not a book for them so I will leave it at that. Protein requirements in the sick and stressed patient also far exceeds this amount, a fact I mention only to show that the one answer solution is usually is ignoring a lot of variables.

How much is enough to help with our goal of long term weight loss maintenance? Once again, it depends on a lot of factors that would be sifted through if you where in my office, including activity level, starting point, etc. I must also keep in mind that if I suggest a level of daily protein intake, it must be high enough to provide the needs of long term weight loss, but not so high that I start implying far too many calories and/or far too few carbohydrates and good fats. The number must also be simple. I know very few people who would pull a calculator out to figure out their protein requirements. It is a balance, but once again, I cannot under-emphasize the importance of protein for long term weight loss maintenance.

I think an adequate daily number of grams of protein for most people to eat, after they have lost the weight and hope to maintain their weight loss, would be approximately 0.8 to 1.2 grams of protein per *pound* of scale weight. Notice the RDA recommendation is 0.8 grams per kilogram. I have simply doubled their suggestion. If you weigh 200 pounds, you need 160 to 240 grams of protein a day to help you maintain weight loss. This equates to 640 to 960 calories in protein a day. If you where to flow into a 1200 calorie a day diet on your weight loss maintenance program, roughly one-half of your calories would come from good quality protein (quality protein I will define in a minute). This, by modern standards sounds like a lot. But as I have emphasized, this is a range not a target. Some days you may get in plenty of good quality protein, some days you may not. That is fine, and part of the solution offered by the Z Diet – it is the big picture we are interested in. If your focus is on good quality, low fat protein, it will also keep you away from those non-essential carbohydrates, one of those subtleties I have mentioned before in the book.

Now that we have amounts, let's define a good quality protein. Quality of protein is more than comparing Spam to Sirloin. My definition of quality protein would encompass all of the following factors: protein content, fat content, carbohydrate content, total calories, speed of absorption, micronutrients, and cost. I had originally written this using headings for each point, but after review, I felt it was too lengthy and had information that would most likely be considered esoteric. So I have simply summed it up for you below.

In my definition of protein content, the amount of a complete protein comes to mind. In other words, a food source with all of the essential and non-essential amino acids available in it. The most obvious source would be animal products as compared to vegetable products. A number of the processed protein sources such as whey, casein, and soy protein powders have an abundance of the branch chain amino acids (BCAA), making them good proteins in my opinion (based on protein content). A number of foods out there are good protein sources, but may have other macronutrients in them that would lessen the total amount of protein. For example, dairy, beans, and nut products are good sources of protein, but due to the carbohydrates and fat that come with them, their total protein content is lower. High fat meats also can increase the not so useful fats in your diet and add considerably to the calories of the protein source - something to keep in mind especially if you are attempting to reach the suggested amounts of protein and keeping an eye on your total caloric intake. With the protein powders and bars, sources of carbohydrates should be considered. These include the high glycemic sources such as corn syrup, high fructose corn syrup, dextrose, rice syrup, maltitol, honey (invert sugar), turbinado sugar, sucrose (which is glucose +fructose), crisp rice, and fructose. Low glycemic sources found in some proteins include sugar alcohols such as maltit*ol*, and lactit*ol*, and glycrer*ol* (glycerine).

The speed of absorption is also something to consider. The processed proteins and protein powders tend to be absorbed much faster and therefore will have a higher glycemic index than something you have to chew or that has fat in it. This comes into play with food timing and your workout or exercise session. Faster absorbing proteins are going to be of greater benefit after a rigorous exercise session, something I cover in great detail in my book **Better Than Steroids**. On the contrary, someone who is metabolically challenged would, in general, be better off with a slower absorbing, lower glycemic protein source.

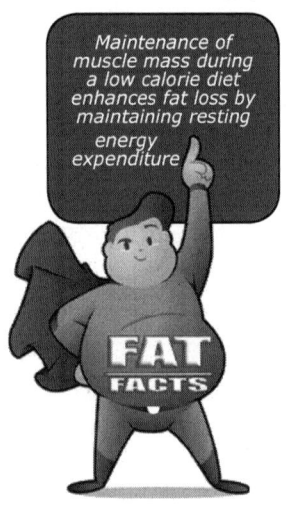

Maintenance of muscle mass during a low calorie diet enhances fat loss by maintaining resting energy expenditure

The amount of micronutrients is also important. Beef and chicken are great sources of iron, zinc and vitamin B12. Cold water fish is an excellent source of omega 3 fatty acids and B12. The protein powders are usually fortified with calcium. Soy products are a source of phytoestrogens that can be of benefit in certain situations.

Cost is an issue as well. In a simple cost comparison of different protein sources available, there is a considerable cost range to consider. Protein such as tuna in a can tends to be cheaper per gram of protein than red meat or other meat sources from the butcher. Of interest, however, is that red meat, which is usually considered the most expensive source of protein, is actually cheaper per gram of protein than yogurt or other dairy products. The protein powders and supplements also have a large cost range. The whey concentrates tend to be cheaper (and taste better, as they have more carbs and fat in them) than the isolates or hydrosylates available in most health food stores.

I am asked all the time "what is the best protein supplement?" so I want to spend a couple of lines on just that topic. Overall, I am a real foods guy. As I mentioned earlier, I would much rather chew my calories than swig them down. Reaching the amount of protein suggested can be difficult for some and that is where I find the protein supplements of great benefit. They also help fit protein into a busy schedule, so when you do not have time to sit and chew your protein, a protein drink or protein bar is a great substitute for the real thing.

I will give you a very brief overview covering, in particular, the most common protein supplements available: milk protein, including whey and casein, egg protein and soy protein. Whey protein comes primarily as whey isolates meaning some chemical processing has taken place to 'isolate' the protein, making it more available to the body. Whey concentrate, also called intact whey protein, is straight from the nursery rhyme (Little Miss Muffet sat on a tuffet, eating her curds and whey) with a little flavoring added. Whey protein has great bio-availability (BV), it is readily absorbed and causes a rapid hyperinsulimic response. It has an excellent BCAA profile as well as being an excellent source of glutamine. Isolates and Hydrolyates of whey (and Soy for that matter) are faster absorbing and therefore better for pre, intra-exercise replacement and post workout. Casein is slower absorbing, as are the whey concentrates, and is therefore better for a night time meal, as a midday meal replacement. It has a slow release effect, as it forms a gel in the gut to slow the transit time of amino acids. Some would argue that this may enhance absorption. Casein also has very high natural glutamine content, and most of the glutamine in casein is found in the peptide form for better absorption.

Egg protein supplements have a great amino acid profile, but their BV is lower. They are very cheap, which is beneficial; however, they have a very well known side effect: You are almost guaranteed to lose friends, family, pets, and your job if you use a lot of this protein... Because of its poor BV, intestinal bacteria getting to this has some powerful effects on your fellow man's (or woman's) olfactory system. Need I say more?

Soy protein is an excellent source of isoflavones and an excellent ratio of glutamine, arginine, and the BCAA's. It is also relatively cheap. Soy, with its phytoestrogens, has the potential to be somewhat estrogenic and therefore has the theoretical potential of affecting males differently and those with hormone sensitive cancers may have to be careful with soy protein. Those with thyroid issues should talk to their doctor before consuming a large amount of soy protein.

All of the protein supplements will advertise vitamins and minerals and additional functional ingredients, but the amounts are of no advantage. Do not include them in your decision to purchase the protein supplement.

Some other important factoids when choosing a protein supplement: avoid baked bars such as bars that contain rolled oats and some granola type bars, as their fat content is elevated and the process of baking denatures some of the protein you are after. In general, the cheaper the protein, the cheaper the protein, i.e. you get what you pay for, but as I mentioned earlier, the whey concentrates are cheaper than the isolated one and taste a little better because they have carbohydrates and fat in them. Hands down, God-made proteins are the best, such as real eggs, tuna, etc. When you set out to buy your protein, base it on the following: What are you using it for? Replacement, Weight gain, Weight loss, etc. You are after the protein, but always look at the calories listed – they add up! Avoid bars with coatings for example. They look the same, but their caloric load is much bigger than bars without coating.

If you are metabolically challenged, whole proteins are best and protein supplements with less than 5 grams of sugar per serving or bar. If you are wiser than most 50 year olds (i.e. if you are 50 years of age or more), protein hydrolysates are best and/or higher sugar content, as it advances the insulin response, particularly before, during, and after exercise.

Fats

Fat is an essential part of your diet, an absolute must in any eating program, and an indispensable ingredient in the quest for optimum health. Not only are certain fats essential in your diet as defined above, but fat in your diet provides an enjoyable texture and an unsurpassed, often craved for taste as well. Removing fat from your diet might work for a few rapid weight loss plans, but it would be this side of impossible to do it on a long term weight loss maintenance program. Fats contain approximately 9 calories per gram. So if you eat 10 grams of fat, you get 90 calories from it. Fat is the most caloric dense of the major macronutrients.

The word fat has a bad connotation to it. It has been unfairly deemed the bad guy and the cause of obesity both in America and around the world. In 1977 the US population was first advised to reduce its intake. It is always with some hesitancy that I say this, but was it not around then that our obesity epidemic started? This recommendation, notably, had unanticipated effects. The introduction of caloric dense sugar based foods with the sales pitch "no fat" or "low fat" has not met the anticipated hope that came with the criminalization of fat. Even in the medical world, data seems to be rather confusing as to the role of fat in disease. The Framingham Heart Study, one of our biggest and oldest studies to date, showed that people with high triglyceride concentrations and low HDL cholesterol concentrations (the good cholesterol) run a significantly higher rate of coronary artery disease (3). Fat intake was (and still is, in many circles) blamed for this; however, the long term health benefits of consuming a low fat diet have not been proven and, to the contrary, some individuals move their risk profile for heart disease in an unfavorable direction by adopting a low fat diet (4). In a study done by Abbasi, et al, 2000, healthy, non-diabetic volunteers consumed diets that contained as a percentage of total calories: 60% carbohydrate, 25% fat and 15% protein or a diet containing 40% carbohydrate, 45%fat and 15% protein. Those consuming the 60% carbohydrate diet had higher fasting triglycerides and lower HDL cholesterol without changing LDL (the bad cholesterol) concentration. The low-fat diet caused lowered HDL cholesterol and included a persistent elevation in lipoproteins. Both of these factors are recognized as important independent risk factors for heart disease and other metabolic diseases.

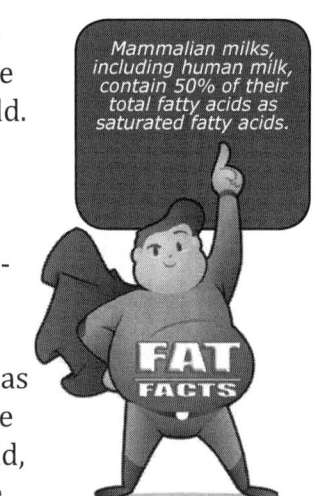

Mammalian milks, including human milk, contain 50% of their total fatty acids as saturated fatty acids.

FAT FACTS

These findings have led many doctors to question whether it is wise to recommend that all of us replace dietary fat (saturated in particular) with carbohydrate. Another example of the "Is Fat Bad" question was The Women's Health Initiative Randomized Controlled Dietary Modification Trial. It looked at approximately 48,000 women to compare low fat diets and increased fruit and vegetable consumption and saw no statistical improvements in heart disease outcomes (5). Disagreement still remains high as to the roles that dietary fat (and cholesterol) play in the risk of heart disease.

The simple answer to this is twofold: 1. We don't know everything yet; and, 2. There are so many variables involved in both health and disease that placing the blame on any one factor alone is ignorant and not well thought out. I could mention an overwhelming amount of conflicting data, but it only tends to confuse me, and I review the stuff for a living. It goes to say that, once again, we do not know everything. Fat has some vital functions in health, disease, weight loss, and weight loss maintenance. I do my best to watch fat intake for myself and my patients, but I try not to criminalize it at the same time.

I will provide you with a quick review of fat. Fats are synthesized by both plants and animals. Fats can be classified into three groups: simple fats, compound fats (made up of a simple fat with another chemical attached such as protein), and derived fats, such as cholesterol, which is a combination of simple and compound fats. Fats can also be classified as Saturated, Unsaturated, Polyunsaturated, and Trans fatty acids. In the average American diet, visible fat constitutes about 30 percent of total fat intake. This includes butter, lard, cooking oils, mayonnaise, etc. The remaining 70 percent comes from invisible fat found in meats, dairy products, vegetables, nuts and seeds, etc.

Saturated fats are found almost exclusively in animal products. They tend to be solid at room temperature. Unsaturated fats can be found a number of places including meat and eggs. They are usually liquid at room temperature. Polyunsaturated fats are found in plants. The omega 3 and omega 6 fatty acids you hear so much about are polyunsaturated fats. Trans fatty acids are more commonly found in man made products, but do occur in nature on occasion. They tend to get a lot of fingers pointed at them for a variety of health problems, but I will simply state, yet again, there are too many other factors involved to blame one or two things for all of life's awfulness.

> It seems that a flat out labeling of fat as bad may be inappropriate. Studies are revealing that different humans with different lifestyles respond differently to fat intakes and to fat compositions. Optimal fat intakes may need to be tailored to individuals.

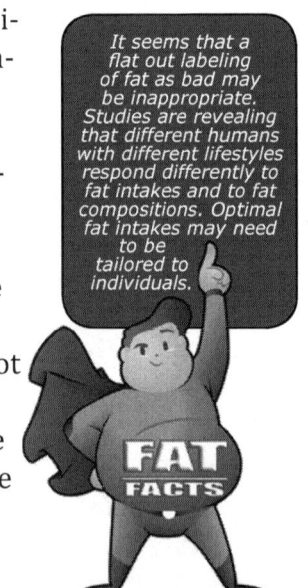

The above is all I am going to cover on the different fats. In general, the Z Diet views fats as an important source of some essential nutrients and an excellent way to maintain some flavor in your diet. Fat does have calories and, as I mentioned above, it is the most caloric dense nutrient. Being aware of your fat intake is essential for long term weight loss maintenance. Your primary source of fat will likely come hand-in-hand with your protein, so consciously choosing low fat dairy, and lean meats is your best bet.

Summary

The basics of food are a must for long term weight loss maintenance. One of the primary concepts of the Z Diet can be summarized as follows: keep adequate protein in your diet, and play/alternate your fat and carbohydrate calories to find the right balance of taste, texture, enjoyment, variety, and ease. This simple technique is a part of the big picture of "how to" maintain weight loss and will be detailed more in coming chapters.

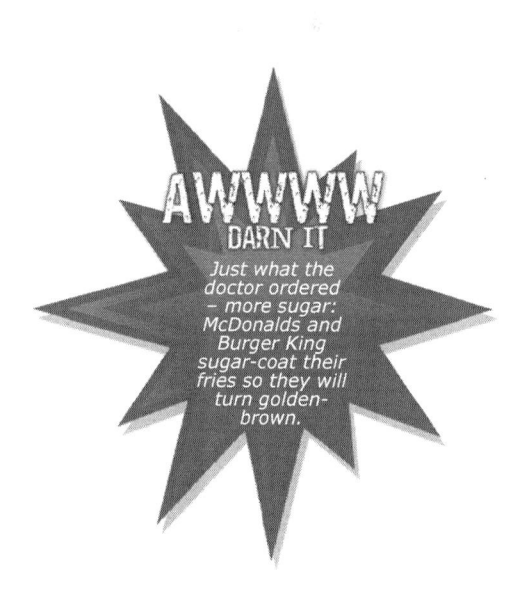

AWWWW DARN IT
Just what the doctor ordered – more sugar: McDonalds and Burger King sugar-coat their fries so they will turn golden-brown.

1. Martin WF et al. Dietary protein intake and renal function. Nutr Metab 2005 2:25.

2. Dawson-Hughes B. Interaction of dietary calcium and protein in bone health in humans. J Nutrition 2003. 133(3):852-854

3. Castelli WP: Lipids, risk factors, and ischaemic heart disease. Atherosclerosis. 124 (Suppl.):1–9, 1996

4. Dreon, D. M. & Krauss, R. M. (1995) Low density lipoprotein subclass patterns are associated with differing lipoprotein responses to low-fat and high-monounsaturated fat diets. Circulation 92 (suppl.): I-155.

5. Howard, B. Van Horn, L. Hsia, J. Low-Fat Dietary Pattern and Risk of Cardiovascular Disease. The Women's Health Initiative Randomized Controlled Dietary Modification Trial. *JAMA.* 2006; 295:655-666.

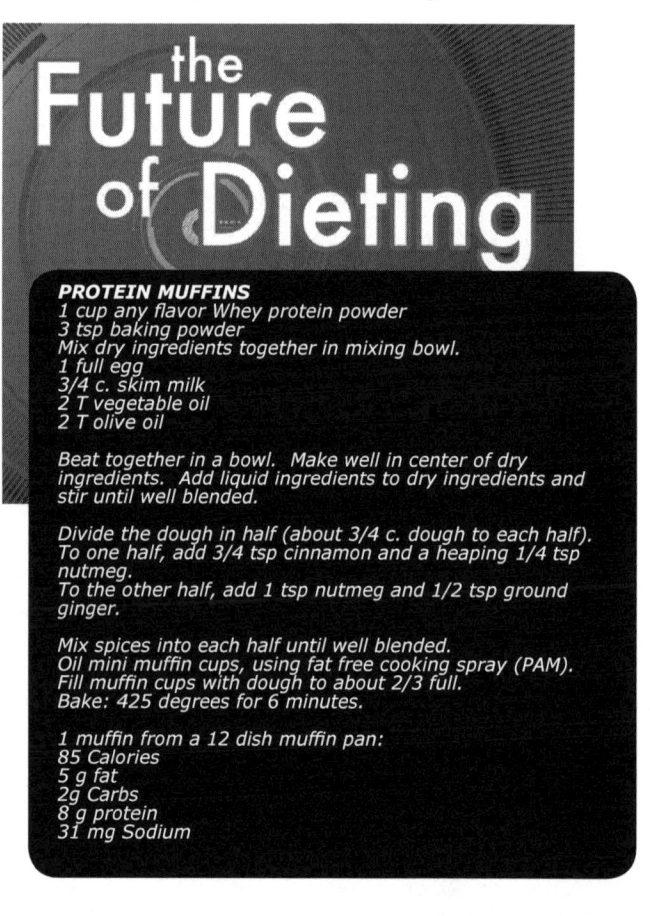

the Future of Dieting

PROTEIN MUFFINS
1 cup any flavor Whey protein powder
3 tsp baking powder
Mix dry ingredients together in mixing bowl.
1 full egg
3/4 c. skim milk
2 T vegetable oil
2 T olive oil

Beat together in a bowl. Make well in center of dry ingredients. Add liquid ingredients to dry ingredients and stir until well blended.

Divide the dough in half (about 3/4 c. dough to each half). To one half, add 3/4 tsp cinnamon and a heaping 1/4 tsp nutmeg.
To the other half, add 1 tsp nutmeg and 1/2 tsp ground ginger.

Mix spices into each half until well blended.
Oil mini muffin cups, using fat free cooking spray (PAM).
Fill muffin cups with dough to about 2/3 full.
Bake: 425 degrees for 6 minutes.

1 muffin from a 12 dish muffin pan:
85 Calories
5 g fat
2g Carbs
8 g protein
31 mg Sodium

4

Willey Principle

As you are more than likely 100% aware, via your own experience, weight loss is attainable with a number of solutions. Weight loss maintenance is a little tougher, as the variables involved seem to increase exponentially. One of the variables I have touched on, and will offer more detail on shortly, is calories. The amount of food you consume is vital. Your portion sizes equate directly to calories, as do the nutrient density and caloric density of foods. The question of calories in to calories out is inarguable, but a number of other factors are also involved. The type of macro nutrients one eats in certain conditions or situations, the amount of processing and artificial chemicals, all have a place, but they are not as well defined. Just as I reviewed fat and its relation to cardiovascular disease in a previous chapter, the number of variables involved in weight loss maintenance is immense and this side of mind boggling.

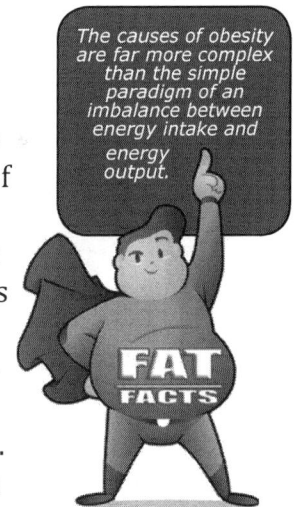

The causes of obesity are far more complex than the simple paradigm of an imbalance between energy intake and energy output.

A number of people will hang their proverbial hats on the side of the argument that calories are all that matter. I have read just as many arguments stating that calories do not matter at all, just X (X being defined as just about anything, for example carbs for the anti-carbohydrate campaigners). Like every argument out there, there are extremes, but the answer usually lies somewhere in the middle. That is why I came up with **The Willey Principle**. It is simply a solution that lies in the middle of the "calories are all that matter", and "calories have nothing to do with it" argument.

The thought came to me as I was helping some patients understand the concept that exercise alone does not cause significant weight loss (I will delve into this in more detail in the Performance section). Just because two things correlate simply means that they are related, but tells you nothing about the direction of the relationship. For example: If X = Exercise and Y = Weight Loss, it is possible that X causes Y. It is also possible that Y causes X (as you lose weight you are more likely to exercise). But more than likely, X and Y are both being influenced by some other factor, Z...

I went digging through patient files, and I went through my own notes for pre-bodybuilding show prep and I started to see a trend. I started to understand some, if not all, of the confusion as to the calories in to calories out question. I started to realize the reason for the discrepancy. In stepping back and looking at both sides, I finally realized something: Both sides are correct.

I then purposely tested it with patients in my clinic – and it was true. From this conclusion, I developed *The Willey Principle*, named of course after the guy who thunk it up!

The Willey Principle states:

- Dependency on caloric load is greater the leaner one gets.

Simply put, the bigger you are, the less you have to worry about calories in to calories out. The smaller or leaner you are, the more calories in to calories out comes into play. To add a little more detail to the theory, *direct* caloric counting and portion sizing become more essential the leaner one gets. If you are extremely large, just learning how to eat with a focus on more quality foods will start the weight loss process. Although the Z Diet was designed for *long term weight loss maintenance*, a number of people use it as their initial weight reducing tool for this very reason. Once they start to lose weight, they will eventually need to monitor their calories with more vigor to ensure continued weight loss or maintenance.

Part of my understanding of the other side was looking at me and those arguing with me. I would assume (slight grin on my face right now) that all registered dietitians and chronic exercisers are leaner, with less fat. If they set out to drop a few pounds of fat, they would have to watch calories in to calories out. They would do this by modifying what they ate and/or they would exercise more – the latter being the easier of the two. All of us in healthcare have to be cautious of the fact that what works for us, might not work for our patients. Hence, the debatable question of calories. If most healthcare givers, diet writers, and personal trainers out there are indeed leaner, with less fat, then of course they need to exercise more and/or eat less, a trait they impose upon their clients. The same goes for me – I am leaner with less fat and if I want to get leaner still, say for a bodybuilding show – I increase my exercise and start obsessing on and monitoring my caloric intake. But I should not expect everyone who comes to my office or reads my books to be the same. Here is where we *both* are correct:

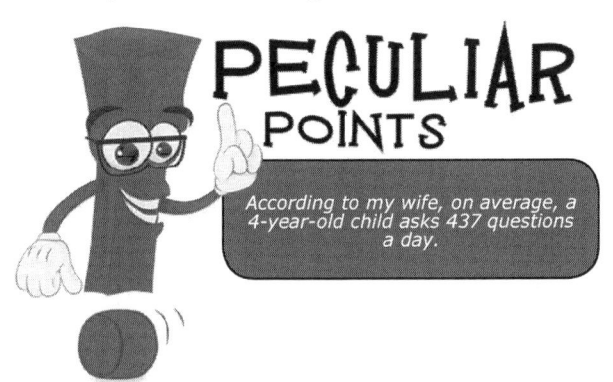

PECULIAR POINTS

According to my wife, on average, a 4-year-old child asks 437 questions a day.

Anyone and everyone in the dietary world would be of the same opinion that larger people have an easier time losing weight at first – operative words being "at first!" There are a number of reasons for this, including the fact that larger people actually have faster metabolisms than smaller people. As a result, *any* change in the larger person's caloric load, direct or indirect, will assist in weight loss.

People come to me all the time for that last 10 or 20 lbs. they cannot get off, and to get it off, I play with their caloric intake. But when a larger person comes in needing to lose a few hundred pounds, I do not initially restrict their calories. I give them the principles outlined in the Z diet (macronutrient shifting, food timing, the *how* to eat, etc.) and they do *wonderfully!* This, of course, can be looked at as *indirect* caloric restriction, but that is ok. It is still working. As they continue to drop fat, build muscle and experience health, I start calculating calories into the equation via increasing output i.e. exercise, or decreasing input i.e. dieting with caloric restrictions. I had unconsciously done this for years, but since I developed *The Willey Principle*, it has become a set tool for use in my clinic – and people do great! This was yet another reason for The Z diet – it allows anyone to lose weight, purposeful caloric restriction or not, based on where they start. If you appreciate *The Willey Principle*, your goals will be easier to achieve.

This brings up another very important concept closely related to The Willey Principle. It is called The P ratio, or Partitioning Ratio. This basically means the leaner you are the more lean you will lose with dieting. The fatter you are, the more fat you will lose with dieting. So when skinny people diet, they lose muscle, whereas when people with more body fat diet, they lose more body fat. The morbidly obese can tolerate lower calories than the moderately obese, with greater retention of fat free mass. This is why The Willey Principle works. If you maintain the style of eating outlined by the Z Diet, you will have an easier time maintaining weight loss. It will also give you some direction to go from your current starting point (something that changes every time you measure). If you are larger, your focus should be on the lifestyle changes outlined in the Performance section of The Z Diet. If you are smaller, apply the lifestyle changes recommended, but also follow your calories a little more closely, as they will come into play with more fervor the leaner you get.

There is a simple fact in weight loss and health attainment that cannot and should not ever be ignored. As a diet writer, health coach, and doctor, the worst thing I can do is torture my patients. Direct caloric restriction and food restriction (types of foods) in general are torture, especially for long term weight loss maintenance. It is one of the primary reasons for dietary failures. I would even go so far as to say they may be one of the primary causes of our obesity epidemic: every solution offered out there is agonizing. Understanding *The Willey Principle* is vital to your success. This book is about maintaining your weight loss once you have achieved it, but you could use it to initiate your weight loss, too. The Willey Principle is built in. As you lean up, get healthier and want to go to the next step, talk to someone about caloric modification. You could also pick up my book **Better Than Steroids**, as it will further delineate eating plans and caloric loads based on lean mass.

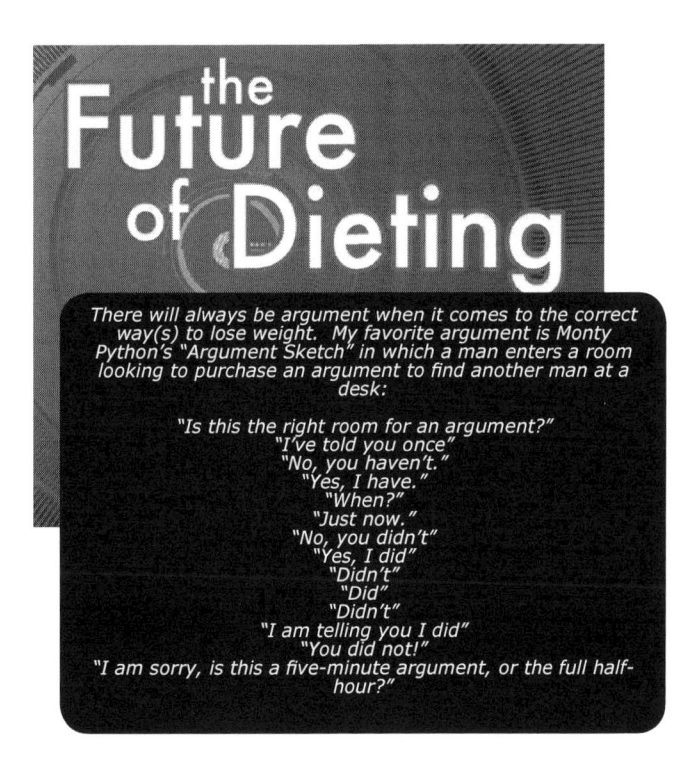

the Future of Dieting

There will always be argument when it comes to the correct way(s) to lose weight. My favorite argument is Monty Python's "Argument Sketch" in which a man enters a room looking to purchase an argument to find another man at a desk:

"Is this the right room for an argument?"
"I've told you once"
"No, you haven't."
"Yes, I have."
"When?"
"Just now."
"No, you didn't"
"Yes, I did"
"Didn't"
"Did"
"Didn't"
"I am telling you I did"
"You did not!"
"I am sorry, is this a five-minute argument, or the full half-hour?"

The Z Diet

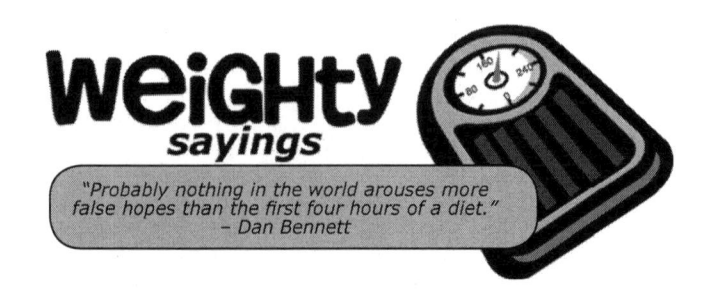

What Happens When You Diet?

Understanding Dieting

Quick Weight Loss Approaches
- Diuresis
- Fasts
- VLED
- LED

WeiGHty sayings

"Probably nothing in the world arouses more false hopes than the first four hours of a diet."
– Dan Bennett

5

Understanding Dieting

The Z Diet is about adherence. It's about sticking to a long term lifestyle for long term and lasting results. Anyone can lose weight; unfortunately, most people seem to find it again. As a weight loss doctor, and for anyone for that matter, it is vitally important to understand why diets are really hard! As I mentioned in the Introduction, the problem with diets is sticking to them. There are a number of reasons dieting is so difficult. When I prescribe a diet, I take everything I am about to tell you into consideration so I can soften the blow in any way, shape, or form I can come up with.

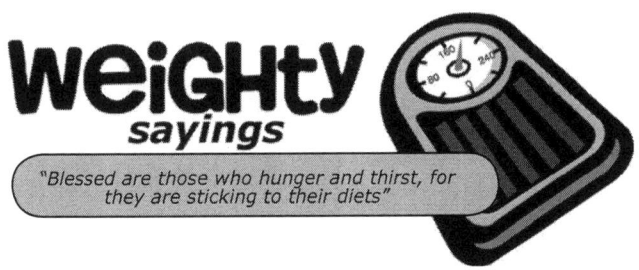

I included this chapter for the simple reason that it is important for you, your doctor, and your loved ones to know what your body is going through when you start cutting calories. Everything I am about to tell

WeiGHty sayings

"Blessed are those who hunger and thirst, for they are sticking to their diets"

you adjusts back to a new found normal when you adhere to the principles of The Z Diet and maintain your weight loss indefinitely. This is also a round-about way of saying "this time keep the weight off"! Your body, your doctor, and your loved ones will all appreciate it! Obviously there is a great deal of science and physiology behind both the positive and negative things that occur with caloric restriction. I am reviewing just a few for you here, focusing on the physiologic and keeping it simple. I eventually talk to my patients about this very stuff in my weight loss practice and therefore I have made the assumption that this is also discussed in most weight loss practices, and consequently is of clinical significance i.e. important to you.

So what happens when you diet? There are obvious positive things that occur, like fat loss, lower blood pressure, improved lipid profile, increase in insulin sensitivity, more energy, etc. You have heard that advertisement also. The negative things seem obvious as well. You feel you cannot have the foods you love, you feel restricted in amounts, you find yourself thinking of food at any sight, sound, or smell that could possibly resemble something you would normally enjoy. You're grouchy, you tend to yell at the kids more than you normally would, you cut your spouse from any remote thought of lovemaking and you tend to slip in to full blown road rage by merely starting your car. Sound familiar? I am sure anyone of you reading this could add ten-fold to the list. The psychological impact of caloric restriction is tough, but it gets worse. I am going to give you a few of the physiological reasons for your anguish in hope of, once again, helping you and your loved ones understand how truly hard it is to lose weight and keep it off. There is, thankfully, a light at the end of the tunnel. All of the physiological things that occur that cause all of the psychological pain return to a new normal, once you have adopted a true long term weight loss maintenance plan like the Z Diet. Please realize that all of these things are related in one way or another. Some of the positives are the direct causes of the negatives, and vice versa.

First, there are the positive physiologic things that occur with caloric restriction. Of course, this is the shorter of the two lists, but I assume you expected that. Your blood sugar starts decreasing followed in short order by your insulin levels. This allows your body to start releasing fat, for energy, from storage sites, such as your belly or hips. Your levels of catecholamine such as epinephrine go up, which increases the fat burn even more. As fatty acids increase, your body starts to utilize them more efficiently, thereby releasing more, and weight loss/fat loss starts to occur. That's it for the good stuff. Now for just a few of the lesser known negatives:

First and foremost, your energy starts to decrease. This is because there is a lack of energy entering your mouth, so your body goes on the fast track to spare the energy you have. This causes you to be fatigued, lack motivation for exercise or even for activities of daily living. You would much rather stay in bed, and that is exactly what your body wants you to do to spare energy. This is part of the reason the most popular weight loss drugs are popular: they give you a little boost of energy because they are all based on amphetamine. Most of the negative physiologic responses I am about to cover also aid in that terrible lackluster feeling one experiences with caloric restriction.

As you cut calories, the androgens in your system, testosterone in particular, increases its affinity for binding to a protein called Sex Hormone Binding Globulin (SHBG). When this occurs, there is much less free or active testosterone available in your system. In plain English, this means all the benefits of testosterone decrease if not disappear completely. A few good things like sound sleep, sex drive, energy, positive attitude, healthy aggressiveness – all decrease or disappear completely. Hence, you no longer want sex and your loved one thinks he or she actually has a problem...you can imagine where I could go from here. Like every negative response I am about to discuss, it is likely a adaptive mechanism. There is no need to reproduce if there is a food shortage. Why bring another mouth into the world to feed when there is not enough food for you?

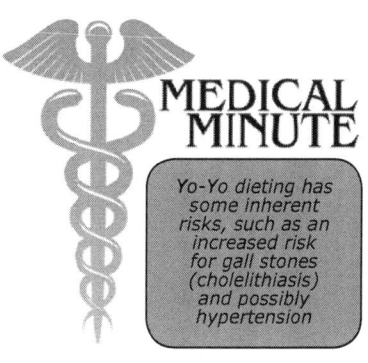

MEDICAL MINUTE

Yo-Yo dieting has some inherent risks, such as an increased risk for gall stones (cholelithiasis) and possibly hypertension

The next problems arise with your thyroid function. I am often told of the many thyroid problems people have as part of their weight problem. Well, thyroid problems or not, when you start your diet, caloric restriction cause a few of its own. With the increased release of fatty acids (a good thing recall), they tend to impair uptake of the thyroid hormone T4 in the liver. That means that even though your thyroid is (hopefully) doing its job and releasing T4 for your body's utilization, the fatty acids inhibit proper uptake of the hormone by the liver for conversion to the active hormone T3. Your tissues also become resistant to T3, causing even more problems. Once again, thyroid hormone functions are beyond the scope of this book, but I am certain you know where to look to find out more about thyroid hormone.

Cortisol, the stress hormone, increases not only because of the obvious stress of caloric restriction, but because insulin, its direct antagonist, is down. Yes, I did mention that as a positive for fat loss, but the negative side of this is cortisol is a catabolic hormone, meaning it has a role in breaking things down, like your muscles. The reasons are many and I am more than happy to discuss them with you but I do not want to have to read a physiology text book here. When your muscles get catabolized due to this effect, you feel it. You are more fatigued, beyond the simple lack of energy you are putting in your mouth. You are weaker; ask any bodybuilder how his or her strength is in the gym on a lower calorie diet. This translates into a real effort to get up and exercise with your diet on the level of the muscles, not your motivation. This negative also prevents the essential branch chain amino acid L-lucine from stimulating protein synthesis and building new muscle, even with all your efforts to do so.

Caloric restriction also causes a decrease in Human Growth Hormone (hGH) and its primary active metabolite, Insulin Growth Factor 1 (IGF-1). Growth hormone is also involved in a number of essential activities in the body, including strengthening your bones, increasing muscle mass, promoting fat burning, helping to balance sugar, and stimulating the immune system.

I will occasionally mention some of the gut hormones involved with the regulation of appetite and satiety, this being one of those times. All of them adjust to changes in calories (too much or too little), but there is one I like to center in on. There is a gut hormone called Ghrelin

MEDICAL MINUTE

Short term weight loss temporarily reduces inflammatory markers such as IL1, IL6, Resisten and TNF Alpha. So if you have sore knees, quit taking Ibuprophen®! Lose the weight!

that skyrockets up in the presence of caloric restriction. You know that deep down, gut aching desire you get when you are hungry - really hungry to the point of being pissed off? That's Ghrelin. You can imagine the negative connotations that brings with it.

The final negative I will cover has to do with your immune system. Have you ever dieted and felt you got more colds and illnesses when you were doing so? Well you were right. Caloric restriction causes your immune response to go down. I have been accused of the perfect business model with my family practice and weight loss clinic being hand-in-hand. I put someone on a diet, which they pay for in the weight loss clinic, and they get sick more often and come see me in my family practice. Obviously, this is not purposeful, but it is the truth. Your immune function is depressed with caloric restriction.

I have covered all of these, once again, to help you see what happens when you restrict calories. All of these physiologic responses are survival in nature. Your body goes into "holy crap" mode and does everything it can to ensure your continued existence. Your body even goes so far as to actually protect fat loss to ensure longer survival with the intention in mind that you will eventually find some food; hence, the decrease in energy, change in hormones, etc. This has one more unfortunate consequence: You have just showed your physiologic body what starvation is like. It does not like starvation, and therefore when you go back to "normal" eating, you are very prone and much more likely to gain *extra* weight, as your body prepares for the next diet...

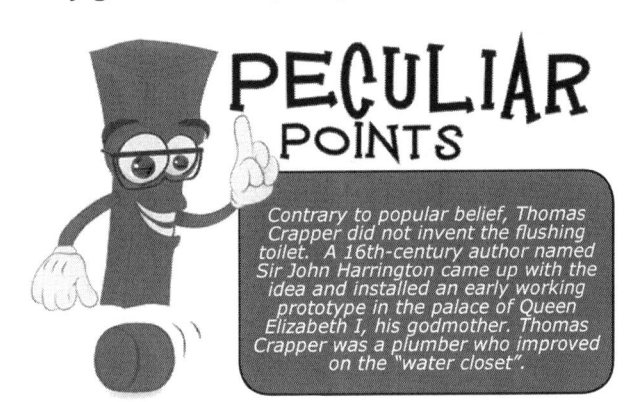

PECULIAR POINTS

Contrary to popular belief, Thomas Crapper did not invent the flushing toilet. A 16th-century author named Sir John Harrington came up with the idea and installed an early working prototype in the palace of Queen Elizabeth I, his godmother. Thomas Crapper was a plumber who improved on the "water closet".

Now for the light at the end of the tunnel: Once you have lost your weight and started a long term weight loss maintenance plan like the Z Diet, all of the negatives just discussed reset themselves and overall, balance back out. The secret is not gaining your weight back and having to go through that again! With long term weight loss you only have to suffer to that extent once. The Z Diet is your solution for avoiding all of those awful things again. Stick to the Z Diet for life and never worry about it again!

6

Quick Weight Loss Approaches

Most, if not all, diets out there are quick weight loss diets. Quick weight loss diets sell because they promise, and in most cases deliver, just that: quick weight loss. They really do nothing for you in the long run other than set you up for quick weight gain, hence – The Z Diet. In my weight loss practice I provide my patients with this information and one if not all of the options I am about to cover for you below, the caveat being – they *have* to sign up for a weight loss transitional plan and a weight loss maintenance plan.

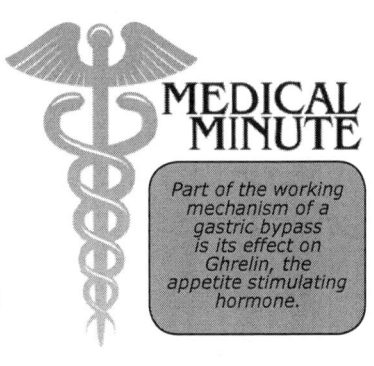

MEDICAL MINUTE

Part of the working mechanism of a gastric bypass is its effect on Ghrelin, the appetite stimulating hormone.

I explained in the introduction how all of these quick weight loss plans work and that the only real secret to their success is the fact that they, in one way or another, by one fancy or not so fancy mechanism, get you to cut your caloric intake, or increase your caloric burn. I am not going to be that subtle here. I am going to tell you the truth from the beginning, including all the ways I am about to review, change your caloric intake. Even more bluntly: all of the ways I am going to review cause you to lose water weight, and cut your calories way too low to survive on for the rest of your life. They are, as the title of the chapter recognizes, quick weight loss approaches.

To sum up the chapter before I really get started, you can use any one of these applications to lose weight quickly. Then you can follow the meat of the book and the Z Diet plan to, at the very least, maintain some of the weight loss you achieved using them. Sound easy? If doing it were as easy as saying it, I would not have written this book.

We will cover four primary ways for quick weight loss: Diuresis, fasting, very low energy diets (VLED), and low energy diets (LED) and provide you with examples of each, as well as review some of the popular plans available out there. In appendix II, I have listed and reviewed a few of the more popular ones with positives and negatives of the plans as well as how they work.

One quick word on safety: Before doing any of these methods for quick weight loss, please visit with your doctor to ensure your personal safety while doing them.

Safety must come first! Weight reducing diets must be *nutritionally adequate* EXCEPT for their energy content. Weight reducing diets should never induce excessive losses of body protein i.e. muscle! Diets should be tailored to the individual, never generalized. *Excessive* weight (in the obese), on average is 75% fat and 25% fat-free mass or lean mass (I will use the terms interchangeably). This combined tissue contains ~ 3200 calories/lb. A 1000 calorie a day deficit will result in 1 lb. Or 3200 calories of acceptable weight loss in 3.2 days (0.3 lb/day), of which no more than 25% should be fat free mass.

If you have ever read any of my other books, or you know me personally, you will be quick to recall one of my favorite subjects in the world is muscle. I like to build it in myself and others; it protects us from disease; it helps us lose fat and maintain fat loss. I do everything in my power to protect it, particularly when people are dieting. Lean body mass loss must be minimized. Lean body mass contains only 363 calories/lb, i.e. muscle is 20% protein, 80% water - For example:

Weight loss of greater than 0.3 lb. per day on a 1,000 calorie/day deficit includes loss of lean body mass. If a 1,000 calorie deficit targets lean body mass, one can lose 2 ¾ lb. per day! This is how a number of the strategies I am about to cover work. If you are not extremely careful, you can lose a lot of muscle mass while dieting. Quality weight loss must be paced! I am reviewing the following information so you are well equipped to understand and sustain long term weight loss.

Three primary factors determine the quality of weight loss: 1. The energy content of the diet. In other words, lower calorie diets tend to cause greater loss of fat-free mass. 2. Macronutrient composition of the diet. Higher protein results in greater retention of fat-free mass. 3. The dieter's body composition when they start the diet. Greater fat loss occurs as the degree of obesity increases for a given caloric restriction (See The Willey Principle).

Most of these approaches should be medically monitored, preferably by an osteopathic or medical doctor board certified in Bariatric Medicine. To find a doctor near you go to http://www.asbp.org/locate_physician.php.

Diuresis

Diuresis simply means the removal of water from your system. This can be done with a change in total calories, as decreasing your total caloric intake causes some water loss; a change in macronutrient composition of your diet (i.e. removing carbohydrates from your diet causes some water weight loss). Other methods include changing the amount of salt in your diet, using herbs, supplements and/or drugs (diuretics).

There are a couple of hormones in your body that are at the primary controls for water retention and/or loss. The hormones involved with this are aldosterone from the super renal glad or adrenal gland and anti-diuretic hormone or vasopressin from your pituitary gland in your head.

Aldosterone and anti-diuretic hormone balance the sodium and water in your body. These two hormones are always discussing ways to keep your water balance in check. If you do not drink enough water,

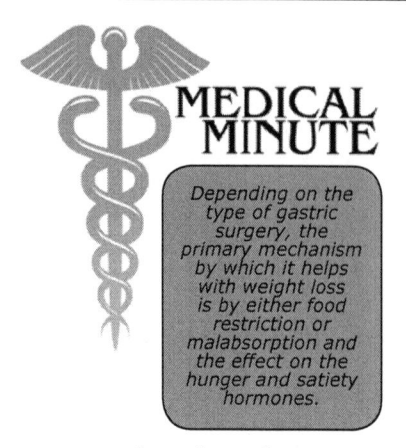

> **MEDICAL MINUTE**
>
> *Depending on the type of gastric surgery, the primary mechanism by which it helps with weight loss is by either food restriction or malabsorption and the effect on the hunger and satiety hormones.*

these hormones cause you to hold on to sodium so you retain the water you have. If you drink a lot of water, aldosterone, an anti-diuretic hormone, allows the kidney to release sodium (excrete it in the urine) and water follows – that is why when you start drinking more, you pee more. Drink less and you visit the bathroom less often. These hormones adapt to your water intake over time.

If you get used to drinking a gallon of water a day, these hormones adjust for it and over time you visit the bathroom less often than when you first started your gallon of water a day crusade. Those of us involved in physique shows use this to our advantage. We will literally water load for a period of time (drink a lot of water for a few days) to change the hormonal interplay and allow the body to get used to excreting excess water as the hormones try to adjust to the increased intake. We then abruptly decrease our water intake for another few days, and in the hormones' attempt to adjust to that change, we continue to excrete as if the water intake was still high and lose a lot of water in the process. This is a very commonly used trick in body building and all of the physique sports as well as in sports where weight class comes into play i.e. wrestling. Adjusting the amount of sodium in your diet also causes these two hormones to fire up in an attempt to maintain a balance. Increasing your salt intake will cause water to be retained (recall how bloated you feel following a nice oriental dinner with lots of salt and MSG) as that balance will be protected. In the same light, decrease your sodium intake and you drop a few pounds of water as your body fights for that same balance.

The simple act of decreasing your total dietary intake will cause some water loss. The first few pounds most people are thrilled to see on the scale when they start a lower calorie weight loss plan are simply the loss of water. Almost all of the diets out there, medically based, fad, or other, have this immediate effect. Low to no carbohydrate diets also have this well known reality, which is part of the reason for their popularity. This water weight loss is short lived, as I am more than certain you have already experienced, as our bodies quickly adapt to the change and adjust by controlling salt and water balance via the hormones in our system. A number of the popular diet plans out there use this to their advantage, including the Cabbage Soup Diet, the Scarsdale diet, and others.

Supplements can also be used to change the water balance in the system and allow for some quick water loss/scale weight changes. These include: Juniper berry (do not use if pregnant, diabetic or experiencing kidney disease), Stinging Nettle, Dandelion, Uvi ursi (bear berry), High dose vitamin C and B6 and Potassium.

The addition of certain foods to your eating plan also helps with diuresis. These foods include: watermelon and watermelon seeds, cantaloupe, tea, apple cider vinegar, celery seed, asparagus, water cress, and cranberries.

A few other things can be used, some of which are considered foodlike substances, to help induce water loss. I have separated these from the above as they need a little more explanation. These include:

>**Caffeine:** caffeine is a very well known diuretic. Unfortunately, its effects are most pronounced in people who do not expose themselves to caffeine on a regular basis. For those of us who are regular caffeine users, or addicts, the diuretic effect of caffeine is minimal. One way to utilize the diuretic effects of caffeine, if you are a regular user, is to avoid it for a few weeks, deal with the headache that accompanies this act, and re-introduce it back into your daily regimen. The re-introduction will induce the diuretic effects of this drug.

>**Alcohol:** Alcohol is a great diuretic. If you have ever had a few drinks and awakened in the middle of the night with the worst cotton mouth

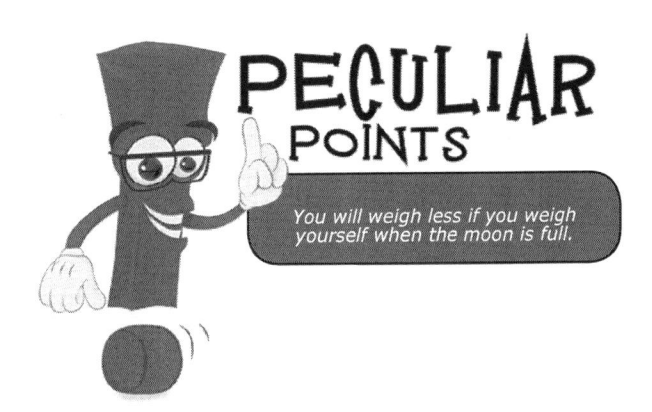

PECULIAR POINTS

You will weigh less if you weigh yourself when the moon is full.

imaginable, you will be quick to agree. This could be of benefit for quick water loss for an event the following day, assuming a hangover is of

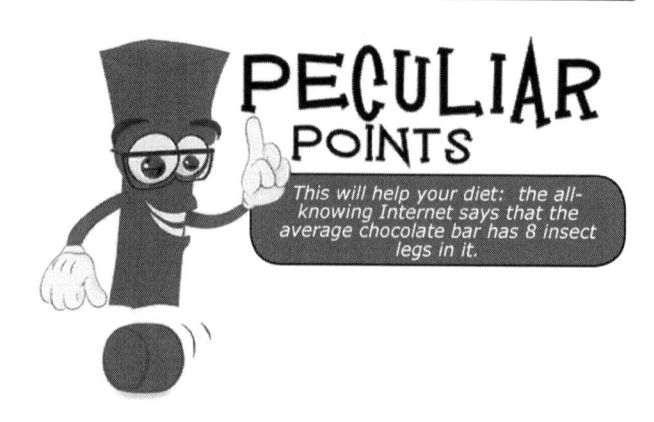

PECULIAR POINTS

This will help your diet: the all-knowing Internet says that the average chocolate bar has 8 insect legs in it.

no concern. Physique artists use this trick all the time. A few glasses of wine the night before an event and you wake up with less water on and in your body.

Extremes of exercise: Working out or sweating out as much water as possible is another way to decrease water weight. This is often used in combination with water loads and depletes, all in the hopes of decreasing water weight.

A few other methods that I really question even mentioning are weight loss body wraps and compression activities that 'guarantee' you to lose inches following a treatment, but since this is a chapter on the quick fix... These wraps will decrease inches, but it is nothing more than water shifting. Good for the short run, no good for the long.

Fasting

Fasting is defined as the complete removal of foods/calories from the diet for a set period of time. Some people may lose up to 20 lbs. over a 24 to 48 hour fast, depending on their starting point i.e. the larger you are or the more you have to lose, the more weight you will drop with a fast (See The Willey Principle). There is some good research on the benefits of short term fasts and many authorities believe there are a number of health benefits related to the occasional fast, including changing insulin resistance, changing leptin resistance, lowering cholesterol, and improving life span. Obviously, the majority of the weight lost during a fast is water and I might have put it under the diuresis section of this chapter. Contrary to popular belief, short term fasting does not induce a metabolic slow down. Some would argue that your metabolism actually speeds up for the duration of a short term fast. Without question, over time or a prolonged fast, our bodies will slow things down to compensate for the removal of energy from the system. A number of popular fasts include additional gimmicks such as "detox enemas" and other various things that fit in different orifices. I am not going to spend any time on these. Certain people should not fast, including: pregnant women, people with wasting diseases or malnutrition, those with a history of cardiac arrhythmias, and people with hepatic (liver) or renal (kidney) insufficiency.

One dietary approach that involves fasting, that could be considered long term, is called the Alternate-day Fast or ADF. ADF's alternate days of fasting (zero food) with days of regular eating. Some studies in mice and other rodents have been very promising in a number of aspects including changes in diabetes risk, cardiovascular risks, and cancer using this method of eating (alternating days of fasting with ad libitum eating)(1-12). However, human studies, however potentially promising (13-15), have not been shown the great results that the little critters showed. This may be simply because the studies were too short, and most of the studies I have read on this topic are done on people of normal weight, and without medical problems - certainly something of great interest as a long term dietary approach. So much so, I have listed fifteen articles that cover it in one facet or another. I have used the technique in a few patients – all did well over all, but I do not have enough information to share with you at this time.

> *A large, 12-year, observational study found that, after weight loss, increases in caffeine consumption were associated with less weight gain.*
> Lopez-Garcia E, van Damn RM, Rajpathak S, Willett WC, Manson JE, Hu FB. Changes in caffeine intake and longterm weight change in men and women. Am J Clin Nutr. 2006;83(3)

Very Low Energy Diets (VLED)

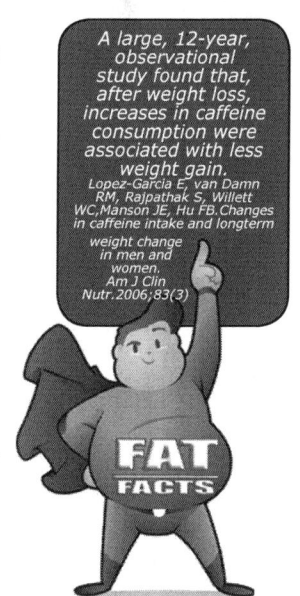

Very low energy diets are also called very low calorie diets (VLCD), and you will see both terms used in the world of weight loss and bariatrics. VLED are controversial due to safety issues as caloric intake is below the metabolic rate of virtually all adults. They do produce an increased rate of fat catabolism. They also seem to decrease carbohydrate metabolism and, very importantly, protein turnover is about the same (high preservation of lean tissue when done correctly). VLED, by definition, are diets with a total caloric intake between 400 and 800 calories a day. These are excellent ways to obtain short term weight loss when utilized correctly. What I mean by correctly is of course, under the supervision of a doctor board certified in bariatric medicine, as it is essential that labs are followed and a baseline EKG is done before the induction of rapid weight loss takes place. One can expect a 2 to 3 pound a day weight loss, once again, depending on the starting point of the dieter. VLED usually consist of quality, lean protein intake to help preserve fat free mass (lean mass/muscle) while on the extremes of caloric restriction. An example breakdown of macronutrients for a VLED is: Protein - 1.5 g/kg of ideal body weight for males, 1.2 g/kg for females (typically 75-105 g/d), carbohydrates - Usually around 50 – 100 g/d to minimize nitrogen loss and ketosis and fat at 10 – 20 g/d emphasizing essential fatty acids. Other nutrients that are needed on a VLED are: Potassium, Calcium, Sodium, Water, Vitamins and mineral supplementation of at least RDA amounts, and Fiber (20-40 g/d).

A number of medically based plans are available through your doctor, including Protein Sparing Modified Fasts (PSMF) and Protein Sparing Modified Liquid Fasts (PSMLF), the Medi-Fast diet, and Optifast.

Some popular ones being used throughout the land include the hCG diet (I will come back to this one in a minute), the Cabbage Soup Diet, Maple Syrup Diet, and The Scarsdale Diet. A few experts in the world of weight loss consider surgical intervention such as gastric banding and gastric bi-passes to fall under this realm - an argument beyond the scope of this book.

As almost all possible examples of VLED lead to the same thing, weight loss via caloric restriction, I will give you a brief summary of one of them, as the comparisons can easily be made with others. All VLED restrict calories, they all tend to differ in the specific "secret ingredient", be it no processed foods, a supplement, or in the case of the hCG plus low calorie diet, a shot. I want to spend a few minutes on the hCG diet as its popularity has, for some unknown tipping point, exploded recently.

The hCG diet (or more appropriately: the hCG plus low calorie diet) is a 500 calorie a day diet that includes the daily intramuscular injection of a small amount of hCG. This diet was developed by a European physician named A.T.W. Simeons and has been around for forty plus years. It goes to show that these diet trends seem to cycle, this one being very popular at the time I wrote this.

hCG stands for Human Chorionic Gonadotropin. hCG is a polypeptide hormone with an alpha and a beta sub-unit produced by the placenta during a normal pregnancy. Its primary role in pregnancy is to maintain the corpus luteum supporting continuous secretion of estrogen and progesterone to maintain the pregnancy. The alpha sub-unit is identical to the alpha unit of luteinizing hormone (LH) and follicle-stimulating hormone (FSH), as well as the alpha sub-unit of human thyroid-stimulating hormone (TSH). Without too many details, I bring this up to demonstrate some of the "secret ingredient" tricks of this particular VLED plan. The similarities of this particular hormone to other hormones in the body provide us with some potential mechanisms of action that I will come back to in a minute.

hCG is not only of prime importance in pregnancy, it is also used in medicine for the treatment of some malady's such as prepubertal cryptorchidism (helping an un-descended testicle in a male child, descend into the scrotal sac), as hormone replacement therapy in males (hypogonadotropic hypogonadism) and for the induction of ovulation. It is also used as a tumor marker (a way for doctors to track, follow, and in some cases identify a tumor). The most well known use of hCG is helping to determine pregnancy. The little stick a gal who thinks she may be pregnant pees on is simply testing for the presence of hCG. If hCG is there, she is pregnant, unless she happens to be using hCG plus a low calorie diet – which will cause the pregnancy test to show positive, without really being pregnant. This can lead to a number of good stories.

As if the low calorie part of this VLED did not cause some body havoc, the hCG portion of the diet, like a lot of the secret ingredients of other VLED, may have potential problems. These include, but are not limited to, side effects such as headache, irritability, restlessness, depression, fatigue, edema, precocious puberty, gynecomastia, pain at the site of injection as well as potential adverse reactions including ovarian hyperstimulation (a syndrome of sudden ovarian enlargement), ascites with or without pain, and/or pleural effusion, rupture of ovarian cysts, multiple births, and blood clots (arterial thromboembolim). The package insert for hCG, as it is only sold as a prescription drug (unless you order it off the Internet, and pray to God above you get what you actually ordered...) even states, in no less terms:

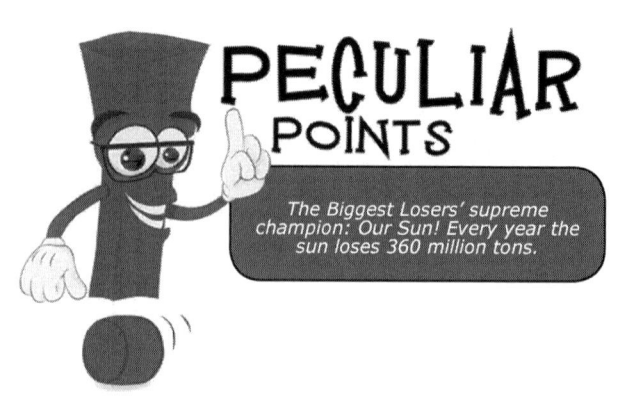

> **PECULIAR POINTS**
>
> The Biggest Losers' supreme champion: Our Sun! Every year the sun loses 360 million tons.

> HCG HAS NOT BEEN DEMONSTRATED TO BE EFFECTIVE ADJUNCTIVE THERAPY IN THE TREATMENT OF OBESITY. THERE IS NO SUBSTANTIAL EVIDENCE THAT IT INCREASES WEIGHT LOSS BEYOND THAT RESULTING FROM CALORIC RESTRICTION, THAT IT CAUSES A MORE ATTRACTIVE OR "NORMAL" DISTRIBUTION OF FAT, OR THAT IT DECREASES THE HUNGER AND DISCOMFORT ASSOCIATED WITH CALORIE-RESTRICTED DIETS.

There is no question that the hCG plus low calorie diet works for short term weight loss. I have seen it a number of times. I have been very impressed with its effectiveness, for short term weight loss. It stays effective when people who utilize it, like all VLED, transition to an eating plan like the one described in this book, for long term maintenance of at least some of the weight lost with the VLED.

Some of the potential theories of the effectiveness of hCG include, beyond that of caloric restriction: The Survival Theory – pregnancy needs to survive to perpetuate the human race, so in cases of starvation (as with the 500 calorie a day plan) the hormone acts to release excess energy from fat cells. The Androgen Theory – hCG increases the production of testosterone and testosterone is a well known fat burner and muscle builder. The Thyroid Theory – because hCG "looks" like thyroid stimulating hormone, it increases the production of thyroid hormone, thus helping with the weight loss. And finally, the Placebo Effect – stabbing yourself in the arm, butt, or leg everyday with a needle is enough motivation to keep you at 500 calories a day.

No matter what the hCG does, or any other secret ingredient with any other VLED plan for that matter, the weight loss attained is what is expected at the total caloric amount given.

VLED should always be done under the supervision of a doctor. I will say it yet again: VLED must be supervised by qualified medical personally! If not formulated appropriately, it may result in generalized protein depletion followed by myocardial intracellular protein depletion (i.e. ventricular arrhythmias)! Those are fancy terms for your heart going into convulsions and your dying. The other problem with them, and the reason you are now reading The Z Diet is the fact that they often result in LARGE weight gain after stopping the diet. Some other potential side effects of VLED are: nausea, vomiting, diarrhea, fatigue, mineral loss, cold intolerance, gout, sagging skin, libido changes, anemia, brittle nails, hair loss, amenorrhea, insomnia, depression, gallstones (up to 25% of users!), anxiety, muscle cramps, etc. People who should avoid VLED completely are persons with diabetes, people in high risk occupations, those with psychological disorders, ulcers, pregnancy, lactation, elderly >65, age <16, heart disease, BMI <30, seizure disorders, chronic use of anti-inflammatory drugs such as Ibuprophen, as well as a number of other medications.

Low Energy Diets (LED)

Low energy diets, by definition, are eating plans that keep total caloric load between 800 and 1200 calories a day. Typically, the macronutrient breakdown is 25 to 40% of calories from protein (1 to 1.6 g/kg of ideal body weight), 20 to 35% from fat, and 35 - 55% from carbohydrates, but these can vary as I will describe below. Deficits of 500 – 1000 calories per day will result in 1 – 2 lbs lost per

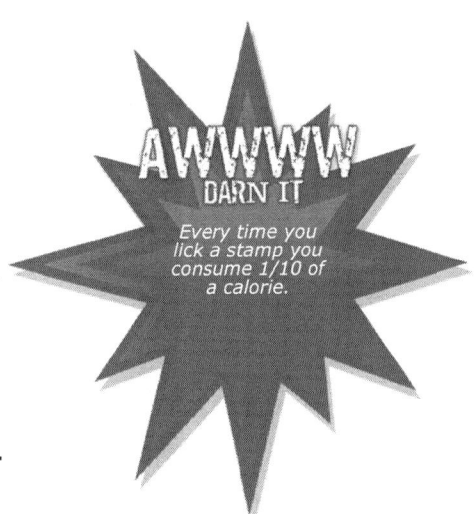

AWWWW DARN IT
Every time you lick a stamp you consume 1/10 of a calorie.

week. The total calories are still lower than most adults' metabolic rates. These diets are appropriate for most disease states as long as they are modified per individual disease state. A weight loss goal of 10% (without exercise) can be expected (75% fat, 25% fat-free). With exercise, weight loss can increase to 20 – 25% of starting weight, if maintained long enough.

Like VLED plans, it does not define macronutrient types or amounts, simply the amount of calories present. In other words, LED can be low carb, high carb, high fat, moderate fat, etc. Unlike VLED, LED's are a little easier to macronutrient shift (change amounts of protein, carbohydrates, and fats) and are also easier in terms of living because one can get away with a lot more on a LED (such as dining out, going to parties, etc.). One of the long term dietary techniques I will cover shortly is called *Diet Cycling*. Diet Cycling involves altering the 'type' of eating plan you are on to help with long term dietary adherence. For example: doing a LED at 1200 calories, low carbohydrate diet for one week, then the following week changing to a 1200 calorie moderate carbohydrate diet, and so forth. For a more detailed explanation, as well as examples of diet cycling options, please refer to my book **Better Than Steroids**.

With the amount of caloric restriction lessened in comparison to a VLED, a lot more variety of foods can come into play. LED can be lifelong eating plans, the caloric restriction being determined by a number of different factors and techniques I will cover in more detail in coming chapters. LEDs fall under quick weight loss plans because the caloric restriction will cause rapid weight loss in some individuals, once again – depending on your starting point. The fatter you are, the more weight you will lose, more quickly, following a LED.

In the next few chapters we will cover some basics that are essential in the quest for long term weight loss maintenance. The information provided is the exquisiteness of the Z Diet. Understand-

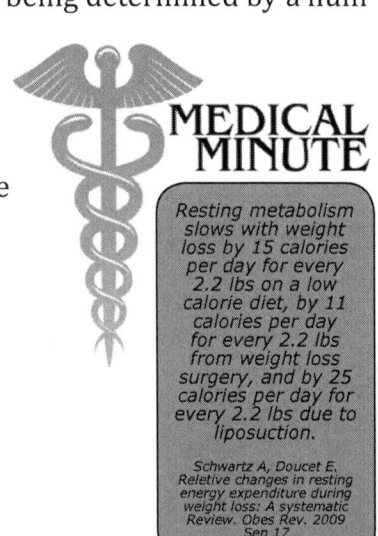

> **MEDICAL MINUTE**
>
> Resting metabolism slows with weight loss by 15 calories per day for every 2.2 lbs on a low calorie diet, by 11 calories per day for every 2.2 lbs from weight loss surgery, and by 25 calories per day for every 2.2 lbs due to liposuction.
>
> Schwartz A, Doucet E. Reletive changes in resting energy expenditure during weight loss: A systematic Review. Obes Rev. 2009 Sep 17

ing and, more important applying, these principles will allow you to maintain your weight loss long term, no matter how you originally lost it!

1. Hsieh EA, Chai CM, Hellerstein MK. Effects of caloric restriction on cell proliferation in several tissues in mice: role of intermittent feeding. Am J Physiol Endocrinol Metab 2005;288:E965–72.

2. Mager DE, Wan R, Brown M, et al. Caloric restriction and intermittent fasting alter spectral measures of heart rate and blood pressure variability in rats. FASEB J 2006;20:631–7.[

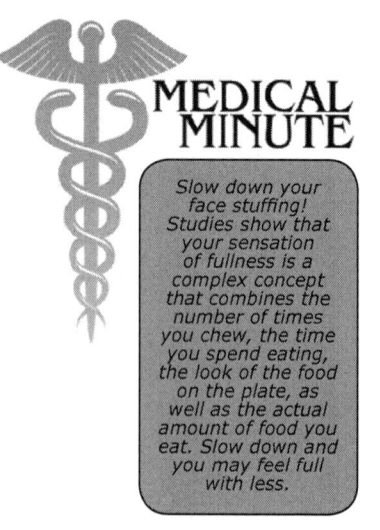

MEDICAL MINUTE

Slow down your face stuffing! Studies show that your sensation of fullness is a complex concept that combines the number of times you chew, the time you spend eating, the look of the food on the plate, as well as the actual amount of food you eat. Slow down and you may feel full with less.

3. Ahmet I, Wan R, Mattson MP, Lakatta EG, Talan M. Cardioprotection by intermittent fasting in rats. Circulation 2005;112:3115–21.

4. Descamps O, Riondel J, Ducros V, Roussel AM. Mitochondrial production of reactive oxygen species and incidence of age-associated lymphoma in OF1 mice: effect of alternate-day fasting. Mech Ageing Dev 2005;126:1185–91.

5. Anson RM, Guo Z, de Cabo R, et al. Intermittent fasting dissociates beneficial effects of dietary restriction on glucose metabolism and neuronal resistance to injury from calorie intake. Proc Natl Acad Sci U S A 2003;100:6216–20.

6. Wan R, Camandola S, Mattson MP. Intermittent fasting and dietary supplementation with 2-deoxy-D-glucose improve functional and metabolic cardiovascular risk factors in rats. FASEB J 2003;17:1133–4.

7. Rocha NS, Barbisan LF, de Oliveira ML, de Camargo JL. Effects of fasting and intermittent fasting on rat hepatocarcinogenesis induced by diethylnitrosamine. Teratog Carcinog Mutagen 2002;22:129–38.

8. Pedersen CR, Hagemann I, Bock T, Buschard K. Intermittent

feeding and fasting reduces diabetes incidence in BB rats. Autoimmunity 1999;30:243–50.

9. Goodrick CL, Ingram DK, Reynolds MA, Freeman JR, Cider N. Effects of intermittent feeding upon body weight and lifespan in inbred mice: interaction of genotype and age. Mech Ageing Dev 1990;55:69–87.

10. Krizova E, Simek V. Influence of intermittent fasting and high-fat diet on morphological changes of the digestive system and on changes of lipid metabolism in the laboratory mouse. Physiol Res 1996;45:145–51.

11. Krizova E, Simek V. Effect of intermittent feeding with high-fat diet on changes of glycogen, protein and fat content in liver and skeletal muscle in the laboratory mouse. Physiol Res 1996;45:379–83.

12. Siegel I, Liu TL, Nepomuceno N, Gleicher N. Effects of short-term dietary restriction on survival of mammary ascites tumor-bearing rats. Cancer Invest 1988;6:677–8.

13. Heilbronn LK, Civitarese AE, Bogacka I, Smith SR, Hulver M, Ravussin E. Glucose tolerance and skeletal muscle gene expression in response to alternate day fasting. Obes Res 2005;13:574–81.

14. Heilbronn LK, Smith SR, Martin CK, Anton SD, Ravussin E. Alternate-day fasting in nonobese subjects: effects on body weight, body composition, and energy metabolism. Am J Clin Nutr 2005;81:69–73.

15. Halberg N, Henriksen M, Soderhamn N, et al. Effect of intermittent fasting and refeeding on insulin action in healthy men. J Appl Physiol 2005;99:2128–36.

The Z Diet

Performance Of The Z Diet

Direct Ways to Control Calories
    Choosing Amounts of Foods
Macro-Nutrient Breakdown
Subtle Ways To Control Calories – LEARN HOW TO EAT
    Biggest Meal In AM, Smallest In PM
    Smaller More Frequent Meals Vs. Other
    Majority of Carbs Early
    Chrononutrakinetics
    Food Timing
    Don't Eat Before Bed
    Energy OUT
    Cyclic Eating
    Scheduled Breaks
    Tracking Results
    When Scheduled; Schedule!
HOW TO Food SHOP and Read labels!
Medications and Weight Loss

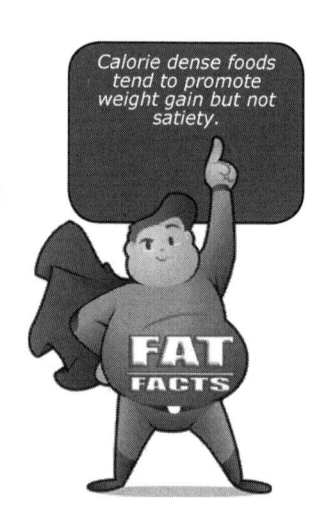

Calorie dense foods tend to promote weight gain but not satiety.

FAT FACTS

7

Direct Ways To Control Calories

This chapter will focus on choosing calories by using some techniques that directly affect the numbers of calories you consume. Once you have lost your weight, it is likely safe to say, you are somewhat familiar with how you feel, when you are hungry, how often you need to eat, etc. These methods will allow you to directly control total caloric intake, *with some forethought*. As is obvious, you could choose to utilize a smaller dinner plate, for example, but still eat twenty three helpings. You will not maintain your weight loss that way. Though not as accurate as directly counting your caloric intake, these methods will work for the vast majority of people reading this. In my continued goal to keep things quick and easy, I will simply state a way to directly monitor your calories, provide a brief explanation, and move to the next.

> Speaking of caloric dense foods: although considered a fiber-rich whole grain health food, commercially prepared granola, with nuts, has more than 500 calories per cup.

FAT FACTS

There will be some crossover between this chapter and the next one on **Subtle Ways to Control Calories**, but I have found if you are consciously aware of these ideas in this chapter, then the more understated ones will add just enough to allow you to maintain long term weight loss. I will emphasize, yet again, the importance of safety when it comes to dieting. Please re-read the importance of safety in the Quick Weight Loss Chapter.

Three primary factors determine the quality of weight loss: 1. The energy content of the diet; 2. Macronutrient composition of the diet; and, 3. The dieter's body composition while he or she is dieting. In the chapter The Willey Principle, I basically discuss number three above. That chapter should have helped you outline a good starting point for your quest for health and weight loss. As a quick review, if you use the Z Diet as your starting weight loss guide, and you are a larger person, do not be so concerned about calories. Just follow the steps outlined here and get your fat moving out of state. Once you start getting leaner, you will have to become more and more aware of your calories for maintenance or to keep moving. If you are leaner, trying to maintain your weight loss from one of the methods mentioned earlier, or attempting to tone up, you need to be much more aware of your total caloric intake. As this book is not for body builders, if you are interested in really dialing in your physique, pick up a copy of my book **Better Than Steroids** for the techniques to do so.

Once again, the other two factors that help determine how food plays a role in your weight loss maintenance are the energy or caloric content of the diet, and the macronutrient composition of the diet, or how much protein, carbs, and fat are in the diet. We will cover each of them separately, but you will quickly see how they all intertwine. As we go through each of them, I will mention distinct areas that refer back to your specific body type or condition so you can individualize your long term Z Diet.

The Energy or Caloric Content of the Diet

While I am certain most of you reading this thinks of your intake in terms of food (What are we having for supper, Dad? My little one just asked while I was typing this very line), I think of it in terms of calories and nutrients. As my little guy asked me that, I arguably and most certainly very nerd like, thought of the number of calories I could have tonight. I was also sure the protein that he and I were going to have was adequate. I think in terms of nutrients and calories not only because of what I do for a living, but also for myself. I keep myself lean year round because I like the way I look and feel when I do. This requires constant monitoring and awareness of what crosses my lips. Why am I telling you this? A number of studies and almost every weight loss doctor out there will tell you the importance of being aware of the caloric content of food. I would also suggest you start thinking in terms of nutrients, which is why I spent the time I did in **The Basics of Food**. I am suggesting you rethink the way you view food. Along with the thought of what is for dinner, think about the number of calories you should be taking in. Recall the amount of protein, carbohydrates, and fats you have had and decide if you need any other nutrients in your diet this coming supper time.

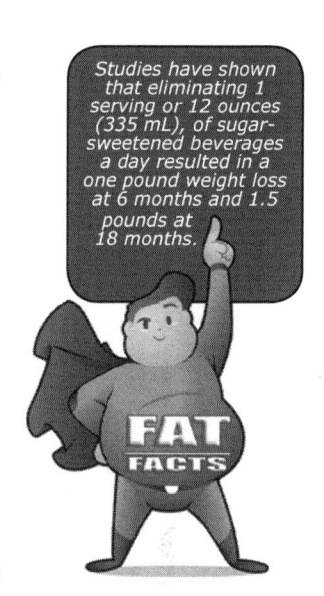

> Studies have shown that eliminating 1 serving or 12 ounces (335 mL), of sugar-sweetened beverages a day resulted in a one pound weight loss at 6 months and 1.5 pounds at 18 months.

Obviously, the amount of food you eat after weight loss is *the* key to how successful you are in maintaining your new found body. For long term weight loss maintenance, your calories must be controlled. Ideally, we would all weigh and measure our food so we know exactly how many calories we are consuming. As I am a realist, I will not insist you do that on a daily basis; however, I am in to portion control and visual sizing of foods, something I am going to explain to you in detail in just a minute here. Before I do, let me say a few words about caloric density.

Caloric Density

By definition, caloric density is the number of calories found in a certain weight or volume of food. Two cups of breakfast cereal have a very different caloric density than one cup of cereal, and one cup of fat free milk. There are two cups of food there, but the energy density of the two examples is very different or the calories per unit weight/volume are dissimilar. Or, as another example, take a bowl of soup. It is full of potatoes, meat, and vegetables, but the majority of it is water, and therefore has a lower energy density.

Caloric or energy dense foods are a primary reason for our obesity problem. It was for this reason that fat was criminalized in the 70s. A few well-respected governing groups of people got together and decided that, since fat is the most caloric dense food type, limiting it would cut calories and therefore help with weight loss, heart disease, diabetes, automobile wrecks, and the middle east crises, etc. Unfortunately, they replaced those fat calories with even more caloric dense processed, sugar filled shit and called it healthy because it was low and no fat.

This is all of great concern in the mission for long term weight loss maintenance. If you tend to eat caloric dense foods, you are very likely to be eating too many calories. There has been scattered research that suggests we each eat a certain amount of food based on weight; if this is the case, then caloric density will have a lot to do with the weight epidemic.

It is simply amazing how many calories a food processing company can pack into a tiny, little piece of "food". For that matter, anything that has been processed is likely packed with calories. Low fat and no fat are no exceptions, so be careful with those. Here is a simple way to look at food: How much air, fiber, and water does the food you are about to put in your mouth have in it? Obviously, processed food has all of the air, fiber, and water removed so it can sit on the shelf and survive a nuclear holocaust. In our brief review of Insulin, we discussed **PFFV** as a way to control insulin's rate of release from the pancreas. Using a similar acronym let me help you think of caloric density: if you wonder how energy dense a food is, think in terms of **PWAF**. **PWAF** stands for **P**rocessing, **W**ater, **A**ir, and **F**iber. If the food you are about to eat has been processed, and or lacks water, air, or fiber – it's likely caloric dense. Avoid it. Another simple way to say that is to eat a lot of vegetables, fruits, and unrefined carbohydrates (lots of good air, water, and fiber in those!). One more example to help you picture the importance of air, water, and fiber and the importance of avoiding processing; compare a cup of grapes, full of air and water and untouched by human hands, and really low calorie for the amount of chewing you get to do vs. a cup of raisins. The raisins are grapes with all the air and water removed, and most certainly processed (almost all of them have added sugar and other chemicals) and the amount of calories…wow! It could be argued that the amounts are the same (one cup) and they are both grapes, but I think you get the point. Being aware of caloric density is a key component to the Z Diet and long term weight loss maintenance.

Caloric density is uniquely different from *nutrient density*. There is really no generally accepted definition for what constitutes a nutrient dense or nutrient rich food, but they are typically defined as foods that provide substantial amounts of nutrients for relatively few calories. Once again, welcome the vegetables, fruits, and unrefined carbohydrates, as well as low fat meats and dairy.

Back to calorie control. You initially need to get a rough idea of how many calories you should be consuming a day to maintain your current weight. There are a number of calculations available to do this, and ones I have used in the past in previous books have been for weight loss, not weight loss maintenance, so I will provide you with a simple one here: Take your current new found scale weight in pounds and multiply it by 8 if you are a female and multiply it by 10 if you are a male. For example:

Female: 150 lbs x 8 = 1200 calories a day

Male: 210 lbs x 10 = 2100 calories a day

This gives you a rough estimate of your total caloric need to maintain your current weight. This *does not* take into consideration your activity level and a few other methods of energy expenditure I will be discussing in the next chapter. This is a simple range for you to use, and make adjustments on according to your activity level, energy, tracking data, etc. I will define that a little more in the next chapter and the section on cyclic eating.

I would really encourage you to spend a couple of weeks and actually calculate your caloric intake, especially now that you have lost the weight. There are a number of food logs on the Internet that can help you do that. After you get a rough idea of the caloric content of your favorite and/or most common foods, you will be able to size up your foods using the portion suggestions listed below. Having a mental image of the amount of food you are consuming is a simple yet effective way to estimate caloric amounts.

There are a number of objects that can be helpful in deciphering normal serving sizes including a deck of cards or a baseball. In the Z Diet, I like to simplify even more by comparing portion sizes to an object readily available – your hand! Estimating portion sizes will get you started toward optimal health and long term weight control.

As you are now all familiar with what a protein and a carbohydrate are, the simplest way to size your food up is as follows: If you are going to consume a protein, including any meat source (chicken, beef, fish, a slab of soy, etc.) make it the size, shape, and thickness of your hand with your fingers all together/touching. Make sure it is low fat, in other words: avoid the marbled meats, high fat dairy, chicken with the skin on, etc.

If you are going to consume a carbohydrate, make it the size of your closed fist. This goes for bread, pasta, cereal, chips, crackers, and any other carbohydrate you have in mind.

I am not going to mention fat here because, speaking in generalities, you should avoid a lot of fatty foods. Focus on lean protein sources, and carbohydrate sources that do not contain a lot of sugar or fat.

Fruit and vegetables fall into the free carbohydrate category. Have as much as you want, unless you are metabolically challenged, in which case stick with the low glycemic fruit and vegetables.

The following is a simple sample of some common foods and the amounts that are appropriate for the majority of people out there. It is only a sample, but you can substitute foods based on type.

1 portion size pasta (½ cup) = ½ a closed fist

1 small muffin = a closed fist

1 portion of cheese = 2 fingers (width, length, and depth) 1 serving of dairy.

1 portion of lean meat (3 ounces) = the palm of your hand (minus fingers)

2 full eggs (scrambled) = the palm of your hand (minus fingers)

1 portion size of nuts (1/4 cup) = an open palm (nuts NOT piled in palm)

1 portion size of carbohydrates such as cooked rice or a potato = a closed fist

1 portion size of fat or oils (1 teaspoon) = the end of two fingers (width, length, and depth)

1 portion size of sweets such as a piece of cake, a brownie, candy = the end of two fingers (width, length, and depth)

1 serving fruits & veggies = 1 closed fist

With your hand as your guide for portion control, here are a few other simple yet very effective ways to help you directly control portions and therefore caloric intake:

The size of your serving dishes

The size of the dishes we use everyday has a lot to do with how much we eat. Start using your salad dish for your main course, and your regular dinner plates for your salads and vegetables. Even better: if you have a daughter like I do (if not, go get one!) use a Barbie© plate that has sections for different foods (like the old camping plates my dad used to have but half the size). They are sectioned out for different foods, and in my experience, excellent serving dishes for kids of any age (that means you!). There are a number of studies that show we tend to eat it if it is there i.e. big dinner plate + big eyes + big portion sizes = welcome back hips! One of the more famous studies was one that used self-refilling soup bowls. This study examined whether visual cues related to portion size can influence intake volume without altering either estimated intake or satiation. The study recruited fifty-four participants in a restaurant style setting. The soup apparatus was housed in a modified restaurant-style table in which two of four bowls slowly and imperceptibly refilled as their contents were consumed. Outcomes included intake volume, intake estimation, consumption monitoring, and satiety. Participants who were unknowingly eating from self-refilling bowls ate more soup than those eating from normal soup bowls. However, despite consuming 73% more, they did not believe they had consumed more, nor did they perceive themselves as more sated than those eating from normal bowls. This was unaffected by their size/weight. These findings are consistent with the notion that the amount of food on a plate or bowl increases intake because it influences consumption norms and expectations and it lessens one's reliance on self-monitoring. It seems that people use their eyes to count calories, rather than their stomachs. The importance of having salient, accurate visual cues can play an important role in the prevention of unintentional overeating. A smaller set of serving plates and dishes is a great way to directly influence total caloric intake!

Order of your food intake: water, salad, vegetables, protein, carbs

Start each meal with a large glass of water, and then wait a few minutes before digging in. Following the drenching of your hunger, eat your raw, bulky, air and water filled foods such as your salad and vegetables that are happily sitting on your bigger dinner plate. After you have devoured those non caloric dense foods, start on your protein source and end with your carbohydrate. This is a very simple yet effective way to help you manage total intake. Take your time to eat as well. Inhaling food does not give

> **FAT FACTS**
>
> Drinking water vs. drinking something else, in particular caloric laden beverages such as pop, fruit juices, energy drinks, sports drinks, etc., lowers total energy intake by eliminating beverage calories. Drinking water vs. drinking nothing at all increases energy expenditure and rates of fat utilization. Experiments have shown that drinking 500 ml of water (roughly 17 oz) increases energy expenditure by 24 calories. Therefore, over a year's time, drinking 1 liter of water a day would increase your annual energy usage by 17,000 calories, equivalent to roughly 5 pounds of fat. Independent of covariates, water is of great importance in long term weight loss maintenance. Most of the studies on this also show something of great interest: non-caloric beverages such as diet pop, diet energy drinks, etc. were not comparable to drinking water, despite similar calorie content. So, once again, Mom was right: drink water!

your gut hormones time to tell your brain you are satisfied.

Dining out

Your best bet is to eat at home, but if you do go out, order from the children's menu. You will get plenty of food, and be amazed at the cost savings. If there is a dish you must have from the regular menu, ask your server to serve you ½ of the dish and bag the second half before he or she brings it to your table.

Know your food

I love to tell the story of one of my patients on a weight loss recheck a few years ago. He and his wife were doing my diet plan. She was doing rather well, and he had made some changes but still needed prodding in a few areas. His wife and I could not convince him to eat more salads and vegetables, so as I walked into the room, I was ready with the question. To my surprise, I entered the room and found him sitting on the end of my examination table puffed up like a rooster on Saturday night. He proudly and without hesitation informed me that he had found "the ideal" vegetable, and planned to incorporate it into his daily eating plan. I, with some regret later, gave him the traditional high five and asked him what this miracle vegetable was. Backing up a little for purposes of the story: My little town in the southeast corner of Idaho had been blessed, or cursed, not a month before this chronicle occurred, with the opening of a Chili's restaurant.

As he remained poised in the cocked position, he proceeded to tell me his vegetable of choice was "the Awesome Blossom" from Chili's. I fell to the floor laughing, thinking he was pulling my leg and knowing the true circumstance of an Awesome Blossom. Much to my chagrin, when I looked up I realized that he did not share my amusement. Straight faced and somber, he said "It's an onion! Good for you, right"?

Estimates you read on total calories being used during exercise are dependent on your weight and your intensity level.

Unbeknownst to him, that particular object of yearning has a colossal caloric load of 2700 calories! Once I shared this with him, he joined me on the floor in laughter.

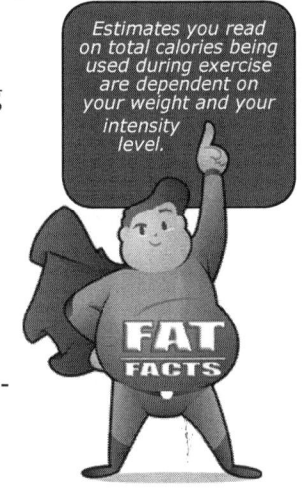

Another classic example of the importance of knowing your foods comes in the illustration from another client of mine, seen at a restaurant. I was sitting at a local steak house with my lovely bride, when I spotted one of my clients sitting at a table not too far from mine. It was obvious he had not seen me, thankfully, as I know how uncomfortable I make some people in public food establishments (not purposefully of course). As I watched him receive his order, I told my wife that I needed to make my presence known, as what he had ordered was most certainly worth some good razzing (I consider all of my clients friends, too). You see, he ordered the half side of beef this restaurant was famous (or notorious) for. I am not kidding; this piece of meat takes two people to carry it to the table! So I got up, approached his table, coming up from behind him on his left side. As he saw me approaching, he glanced over his left shoulder and without hesitation said "hey doc! Good to see you! Look what I got!" As I glared down at his plate, I realized he had cut that hunk of beef into three equal pieces. He proceeded to tell me that every time I wrote a piece of red meat on his eating plans, they approximated 1/3 of the slab he had on his plate. He had already taken the liberty of cutting it up; one piece now, and the other two for a later date. Without difficulty, he knows his food!

Knowing your food is an essential part of long term weight loss maintenance. Take time to look at labels (see How to Shop and Read Labels), and ask for a nutrient breakdown from your favorite restaurant. You may be amazed at what you have been eating! Knowing your food will help you control what you will be eating in the future.

Avoid Liquid Calories

By 2004, Americans were consuming over 135 gallons of fluid other than water every day (about 1.5 liters/person). Beverages sweetened with High Fructose Corn Syrup are consumed at a rate of 35 gallons/year, (followed by beer consumption...which at least has some nutrients...). Globally, 1 billion soda drinks are swallowed each day, including energy drinks. Now, that is a lot of calories. But it is a lot more than just a calorie problem. Let me clarify: it is a calorie problem, but there is a lot more going on than meets the eye.

Let's back up a few hundred thousand years and discuss what our great, great, great, great grandfathers drank. They drank water, water, and then they had some water, and occasionally milk. That's it. Water is of course water, a wonderful calorie free beverage that you will certainly die without – 'nuff said. Milk contains protein, carbs, fat, vitamins, etc. and by some is considered 'food'. This is important in considering something called caloric compensation. Caloric compensation in dietary terms is the adjustment of the body to calories consumed throughout the day. This means, back to that regulatory, homeostatic mechanism at play, that if you sit down at lunch and eat 1500 calories, you are likely to eat less food later in the day, as you have compensated for the load at lunch. Unfortunately, when you drink 1500 calories in pop in a day, a number of studies show that we humans *cannot* compensate for the liquid calories. Why? I will mention a couple reasons, but I won't dive too deep here: Evolutionarily speaking, we never developed the ability, as sugar/caloric filled beverages are rather new on our human time line. Second, liquid calories are absorbed too quickly for hormonal reparation. Your hormones never have a chance to respond to the calories and tell your brain you have had enough.

What does this all mean? The intake of liquid calories (primarily sweetened drinks) does *not* reduce your intake of solid food! Some studies have even shown an *increase* in calories consumed in solid food with sweetened beverages in your diet! Why is this country fat again?

Wait! There is more! Sensory mechanisms respond differently to things in solution vs. solids. This means that when something tastes good in solid form, it is much better in liquid form. Your taste buds respond to them differently! Sweet beverages are sweeter than solid sweets. Even the smell of sweet liquids (even diet drinks…) increases the cephalic insulin response. That means when you smell something sweet like that sugar-filled, told it's good for you, fruit juice or soda pop, you get hungry and tend to eat to satisfy it.

Simple physics even provides some clues: Pour a liquid down a tube vs. pouring some mud down a tube. Your body literally does not see the sodas, fruit juices, and energy drinks until the calories are absorbed in the small intestine. The hormonal guards that tell you to quit stuffing your gullet never had time to respond!

What about alcohol? This one is a little more interesting. It seems that drinking a lot of alcohol causes weight to go up in men, but stay the same or go down in women.

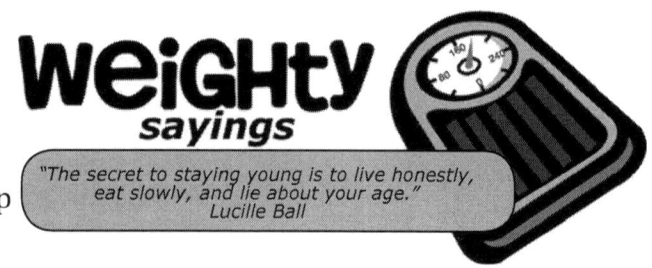

weiGHty sayings

"The secret to staying young is to live honestly, eat slowly, and lie about your age."
Lucille Ball

This is most likely due to the fact that the guys get together and drink beer, then order pizza and wings, while the gals are a little more conscious and just have a drink or two, without the accompanying large influx of food. There is some research that points out that regular drinkers may be more active than their non-drinking counter parts, yet another argument for a different stage. In summary: other than the occasional low fat milk, avoid liquid calories at every turn. I personally would much rather chew my calories than drink them.

Summary

These are some simple methods for you to put in place on the Z Diet to directly influence your total caloric intake. You are likely to cuss at me for saying it yet again, but your best bet is to actually count your calories out and make adjustments based on tracking changes. In the next short chapter I will make some macro nutrient suggestions based on the four classifications I mentioned earlier in the book. The following chapter contains a number of methods to help you indirectly control your total caloric intake, as well as mention the ways your body burns calories. Understanding the direct methods used to count calories, choosing the appropriate macronutrient breakdown, and living according to the life style of the Z Diet with subtle caloric control, you will find it a lot easier to enjoy the benefits of long term weight loss maintenance.

1. Wansink B. Painter JE. North J. Bottomless bowls: why visual cues of portion size may influence intake. Obes Res. 2005. Jan:13(1):93-100

8

Macro-Nutrient Breakdown

I am purposely keeping this chapter short, as it actually has the potential to be very big. I have to keep it undersized, to prevent me from rambling. I am going to provide you with simple ways to figure out how many carbohydrates and how much fat you need a day to maintain your weight loss. I will refer back to the body categorization chapter for definitions of each heading. The surrounding chapters have to do with calories, so I will just briefly mention them here.

A number of studies indicate that macronutrient modification is a more powerful tool in fat loss, particularly abdominal fat, than low fat calorie restricted diets.

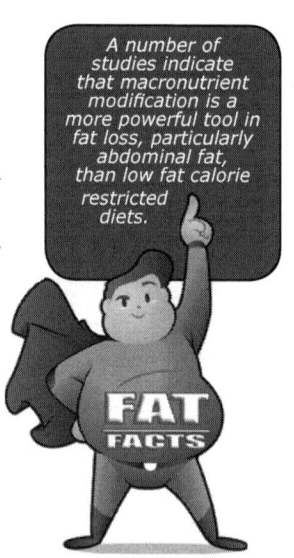

As we discussed in Basics of Food, it is essential in long term weight loss maintenance to keep your protein intake high, or at least higher than you used to. This is one calculation you must do, because you can guess the amounts of carbohydrates and fats you will need to consume after you derive the protein amount. I think an adequate number of grams of protein for most people to eat a day after they have lost the weight and hope to maintain their weight loss, would be approximately 0.8 to 1.2 grams of protein per *pound* of scale weight. If you weigh 200 pounds, you need 160 to 240 grams of protein a day to help you maintain weight loss. This equates to 640 to 960 calories in protein a day. If you were to flow into an 1800 calorie a day diet on your weight loss maintenance program, roughly one-third of your calories would come from good quality protein. By modern standards this sounds like a lot, but as I have emphasized, this is a range not a target. Some days you may get in plenty of good quality protein, some days you may not. That's OK. Remember, choose lean meats, avoid processed proteins when you can, and use protein supplements when and where they're needed. Once you have determined the amount of protein you need, you need to equate that to real food. I have provided a chart below to help you do that. This will give you the comparisons you need to figure out how much protein it will take to get to your suggested amounts. Be sure to spread protein out over your entire day, be it three meals or six – every time you eat you should be consuming some protein.

As far as carbohydrates go do the following: Fruit and vegetables fall into the free carbohydrate category. Have as much as you want, unless you are metabolically challenged, in which case stick with the low glycemic fruit and vegetables. In Appendix I there is a list of the lower glycemic fruits to pick from. As for the active carbohydrates, be smart in your selection. There is no such thing as a bad food, remember? Use the suggestions throughout the Z Diet to achieve the right amounts. Keep in mind real the Z Diet is a *lifestyle*. Your lifestyle waxes and wanes with your activity, stressors, days, weeks, months, etc. This is merely providing a framework. If you are a heavy exerciser or have a strenuous day, your active carbohydrate need may increase. Let it! The big picture of long term weight loss management is what we are focusing on!

Our discussion of the macronutrient fat is just as simple: avoid it. Pick the fat free version of everything you purchase, but keep a keen eye on sugar content and total calories! I have provided a way to view labels in a coming chapter so refer to that often. Remember: the Z Diet is about a simple way to maintain the weight loss you have achieved.

The Metabolically Challenged

If you are metabolically challenged and you are on the larger side (% body fat >35 if you are female and > 25 if you are male), you have a lot more room to play with calories and will most certainly do best with a *no to low* active carbohydrate diet. This would be similar to the Keto run diets I discuss in **Better Than Steroids**, with scheduled breaks or free windows (see the next chapter) every few weeks.

If you are smaller (% body fat > 22 if you are female and > 15 if you are male) you need to be more concerned about your caloric intake, and you too will certainly do best to keep your active carbohydrate content/amount low. This can be accomplished with a lower carbohydrate diet. In the design of the Z Diet, this means you would calculate your protein at the maximum amount suggested (scale weight in pounds multiplied by 1.2) to get the number of grams needed a day of protein. Then eat some low glycemic carbohydrates for breakfast in the amount suggested in the previous chapter, using your hand as your reference, and ½ that amount midday, and then do your best to avoid active carbs the rest of the day. As your body recovers from its insulin predicament, start adding more carbohydrates throughout the day.

The Hormonally Challenged

Balancing hormones, in particular the thyroid and sex hormones, is very beneficial for long term weight loss maintenance, something you should see your doctor for if you are concerned you have a problem there. In men, low testosterone or Andropause can cause a world of problems and difficulties that most certainly can be avoided. A simple way to tell if you might have low testosterone is if you are in your late thirties or beyond and your belly is bigger than your chest, have your doctor run a blood test. Of course, this could be a beer and pizza problem, but the chicken and the egg question will not be mentioned here. I would also suggest you pick up a copy of my book **What Does Your Doctor Look Like Naked?** and fill out the ADAM Questionnaire in the chapter on male hormone replacement. If your gut is larger than your chest, and you answer the ADAM questionnaire in the positive, see your doctor.

Women who are hormonally challenged have a lot more going against them, as I am sure the gals out there reading would be quick to agree. I want to cover a few things here before I make the simple macronutrient suggestion. Again, doing my best to spare you esoteric information and get right to the take home point: Estrogen gets unfairly blamed for fat gain, all too commonly for a woman's fat, particularly fat on the lower extremities.

> A simple dietary intervention, with the sole focus on the promotion of drinking water, effectively reduced the incidence of overweight among school children.
> Muckelbauer, R. Libuda, L. Clausen, K. A Simple Dietary Intervention in the School Setting Decreased Incidence of Overweight in Children. Obes Facts 2009;2:282-285

If you look at a women's menstrual cycle, studies show that when estrogen is at its highest right before ovulation (mid-cycle) energy intake is actually decreased (i.e. you eat less). Women tend to eat less during the Follicular Phase (the first day you menstruate to mid-cycle and ovulation) of the menstrual cycle, and start eating a lot more during the second half of the menstrual cycle called the Luteal Phase when estrogen is decreasing. Estrogen appears to improve Leptin signaling in the brain, or at least send a leptin-like signal to the brain. Leptin is the hormone released from the fat cell telling your brain you are full.

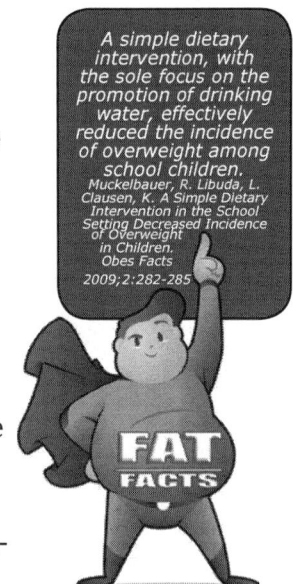

After ovulation in the luteal phase, estrogen starts to decrease and progesterone starts to rise. This causes an increase in energy expenditure i.e. you burn more calories in the luteal phase of your cycle. During this time is when most gals will admittedly crave high fat and sugar dense foods such as chocolate. So like all of life's other equality, in the luteal phase of the menstrual cycle your metabolism increases and so does your eating! This increase in caloric expenditure is roughly 3 to 11% and equates to roughly 90 to 300 calories, but the average intake of food increases by 90 to 500 calories. You tend to make up for it and then some. It is difficult to say if this is due to the falling estrogen, or the increase in progesterone. I would be one to argue it is likely due to both, because nothing is ever simple.

Understanding this is essential in the Z Diet and long term weight loss maintenance for a couple of reasons: first, never start a diet before your menstrual cycle begins – you are more likely to fall off of it due to the increased need for calories. On a brighter note, if you are able to handle the pressure, you will lose more weight at this time if you keep your calories under control as your metabolism is running faster (told you nothing was ever simple!). Second: if your menstrual cycle is off i.e. you are peri-menopausal or menopausal, a doctor comfortable with hormone replacement therapy may help you to regulate it and therefore derive the benefits in your long term weight loss maintenance. And finally: Almost universally when I ask the wonderful gals I work with in my clinical practice what they crave before their cycle starts, their response is a resounding 'chocolate'. As I just mentioned, high fat and sugar dense foods are what are craved the most, and chocolate meets that criteria. Chocolate is also one of the highest natural sources of magnesium, and a few studies point out that this nutrient may be what is sought after during that time of the month. Purely from an analogy stand point, it's kind of like a salt lick in a pasture for the cows (really – no offense there!). As part of your long term weight loss goals, hormonally challenged or not, taking 400 mg of magnesium every night might be of great benefit in keeping calories under control pre-menstrually.

As to the macronutrients, if you are hormonally challenged and you are on the larger side (% body fat >35 if you are female and > 25 if you are male.), you have a lot more room to play with calories and will most certainly do best with a low active carbohydrate diet alternating with a high carbohydrate, moderate fat diet – something I call a Modified Carb Drop (MCD). This is done by calculating your protein requirements to reach your minimum for the day and alternating days of higher and lower carbohydrates in a controlled fashion. The best way to do this for someone hormonally challenged with the body compositions mentioned above is to alternate five days of low carbohydrate eating, followed by a day or two of higher carbohydrate eating and repeat. This works well as a lifestyle plan with the Z Diet because you can alternate your high and low carbohydrate days based on your weekly and weekend schedule or activity level. Weekends are not as controlled and we are more likely to frequent parties and eat out, so raising your carbohydrates on these days fits in nicely.

If you are smaller (% body fat >22 if you are female and > 15 if you are male) you need to be more concerned about your caloric intake and therefore it would be wise to calculate calories and really plan ahead. The style of eating would be the same as for the larger folks in this category, using a MCD and alternate low active carbohydrate diet alternating with a high carbohydrate diet but alternate it more frequently. For example: Calculate your protein content, avoid fat where you can, and eat a lower carbohydrate diet for two of three days in a row, then have one higher carbohydrate diet day, and repeat it (go back to the low carb diet for a few days). Please refer to the next chapter and the portion that discusses cyclic dieting and my book **Better Than Steroids** for more detail.

The Physique Oriented

The Physique Oriented person is someone of average risk without medical problems or concerns whose primary goal is physique development. This means they do not have metabolic or hormonal concerns, as defined above, when they set out for their long term maintenance plan. If you are larger when you start this approach (percent body fat greater than 25 for a male and 30 for a female), check with your doctor for some lab work and an evaluation to be sure you do not fall into the metabolically challenged category. You could also take the Insulin Questionnaire for a little direction.

As far as lasting eating plans, cyclic eating is essential as well as keeping a *very* close eye on calories and adjusting them according to your body's changes, the amount of cardio you are doing, etc. A simple starting place for the physique oriented person is (obviously) getting enough protein in the diet as well as an adequate amount of carbohydrates, based on the amount of activity and exercise he or she is doing. Applying the principles of the Z Diet will most certainly help in your body morphing goals, especially when you tighten up your calories for that last few pounds, or that dress size that is just evading you.

As a reiteration: the physique oriented person differs in a few key areas in long term weight loss maintenance in the sense that vigorous exercise must be a part of his or her daily regimen. Exercise plans are beyond the scope of this book, but I have a number of sample plans available for download on my website www.eatright4u.com.

General Health

The classification for the person who recently lost weight and wants to maintain it for life, whose is not metabolically challenged, does not have hormonal issues, and does not have a lot of physique goals other than never gaining their weight back, fall into this category. In my experience, this could apply to anyone who has found successful weight loss, but now need a way to keep it off. Simply put; the Z Diet *is* your answer to long term weight loss. Calculate your daily protein amounts, use the ideology in the Z Diet, and keep that weight off!

Summary

In the last chapter I reviewed direct ways to watch caloric intake, specifically, in regard to the macronutrients, using your hand size as a determinant of portion sizes. Let me quickly review: Protein portions should be the size, shape, and thickness of your hand with your fingers all together/touching. Make sure it is low fat; in other words, avoid the marbled meats, high fat dairy, chicken with the skin on, etc. If you are going to consume a carbohydrate, make it the size of your closed fist. This goes for bread, pasta, cereal, chips, crackers, and any other carbohydrate you have in mind. I am not going to mention fat here because, speaking in generalities, you should avoid eating a lot of fatty foods. Avoid processed foods and focus on lean protein sources, and carbohydrate sources that do not contain a lot of sugar or fat and are not energy dense - remember **PWAF** (**P**rocessing, **W**ater, **A**ir, and **F**iber). Fruits and vegetables fall into the free carbohydrate category. Have as much as you want, unless you are metabolically challenged, in which case stick with the low glycemic fruit and vegetables.

The 'average' hand is equivalent to about four ounces of cooked meat and one cup of a few other common proteins available. Seed, nut, and bean amounts would encompass an open handful. I have provided the following chart for comparisons of different protein sources, amounts in grams and calories. If you are the math type and recall that I told you that one gram of protein has four calories in it, you will be quick to notice that the grams and calories do not add up. The reason is I did not include carbohydrates or fat calories in the food sources. These, I consider primary proteins and therefore the fat and carbohydrates of course count in the total calories (that is why I listed the total calories), but the only calculation I asked you to do was the amount of protein in grams based on your scale weight. It would serve you well to choose a protein source with a lower caloric amount as this simply means calories from fat and carbohydrates are fewer.

Protein Source	Serving Size		Calories	Grams Protein
1% cottage cheese	1	Cup	160	24
2% cottage cheese (low fat)	1	Cup	200	30
Cottage cheese (fat free)	1	Cup	160	28
Cottage Cheese Dry Curd	1	Cup	105	24
Bass, Freshwater, Dry Heat	4	Oz	165	28
Bass, Striped, Dry Heat	4	Oz	140	25
Cheddar, Shredded, Fat Free,		Cup	45	10
Cheddar, Shredded, 94% Fat Free		Cup	50	8
Cheese, Colby/Mozzarella	4	Oz	440	28
Mozzarella Shredded, Fat Free		Cup	50	9
Chicken Breast (Hormel/Can)	1	Can	150	30
Chicken Breast (Skinless)	4	Oz	120	26
Chicken (Leg W/ Skin & Bone)	1		265	30
Chicken (Thigh W/ Skin & Bone)	1		153	16
Chicken (Leg & Thigh W/ Skin & Bone)	1		418	45
Cod, Atlantic, Dry Heat (Dry Heat)	4	Oz	119	25
Crab, Alaska King, Moist Heat	4	Oz	109	23
Crab, Blue, Moist Heat	4	Oz	116	23
Egg White	3		51	11
Egg, Whole	3		225	20
Egg Beaters	1	Cup	120	24
Flounder, Dry Heat	4	Oz	132	28
Haddock, Dry Heat	4	Oz	127	28
Halibut, Dry Heat	4	Oz	159	31
Ham 96% Fat Free	4	Oz	140	18
Ham, Dark Meat, Canned	4	Oz	120	20
Hamburger, (10 % Fat)	4	Oz	225	29
Hamburger, (15 % Fat)	4	Oz	272	29
Hamburger, (20 % Fat)	4	Oz	280	20
Hamburger, (27 % Fat)	4	Oz	331	27
Lamb, Shoulder	4	Oz	352	14
Lobster, Northern, Moist Heat	4	Oz	111	23
Mahi Mahi	4	Oz	97	21
Orange Roughy, Dry Heat	4	Oz	101	21
Perch, Dry Heat	4	Oz	132	28
Perch, Ocean/Atlantic, Dry Heat	4	Oz	137	28

Protein Source	Serving Size		Calories	Grams Protein
Pork, Sirloin, Lean W/ Fat	4	Oz	400	25
Salmon, Atlantic, Dry Heat	4	Oz	208	29
Shrimp, Moist Heat	4	Oz	112	24
Steak, Bottom Round	4	Oz	237	36
Steak, Brisket (Flat Half)	4	Oz	252	36
Steak, Chuck, Arm	4	Oz	244	37
Steak, Chuck, Blade	4	Oz	284	35
Steak, Eye Round	4	Oz	191	33
Steak, Flank	4	Oz	235	31
Steak, New York Strip	4	Oz	200	30
Steak, Porterhouse	4	Oz	247	32
Steak, Rib Eye	4	Oz	255	32
Steak, Round Tip	4	Oz	209	35
Steak, Shank (Crosscuts)	4	Oz	228	39
Steak, T-Bone	4	Oz	243	32
Steak, Tenderloin	4	Oz	239	31
Steak, Top Loin	4	Oz	235	32
Steak, Top Round	4	Oz	204	36
Steak, Top Sirloin	4	Oz	220	35
Steak, Tyson Seasoned Beef Strips	4	Oz	187	27
Taco/Burrito Meat/Smart Ground	1	Cup	192	30
Trout, Dry Heat	4	Oz	215	31
Tuna, Low Sodium, Canned	1	Can	175	39
Tuna, Water, Canned	1	Can	150	32
Tuna, White / Lo Salt, Can (1 Can / 5 Oz)	1	Can	175	37
Tuna, White, Can (1 Can / 5 Oz)	1	Can	175	40
Tuna, Fillet/Steak	4	Oz	176	32
Turkey Breast (Skinless)	4	Oz	214	32
Turkey Breast (Canned)	1	Can	175	28
Turkey Brst/Oven Roast - 89% Ff	4	Oz	100	16
Venison / Antelope	4	Oz	179	34
Walleye	4	Oz	135	28
Almonds	1	Oz	170	6
Michael Angelo Lasagna W/ Meat	1	Cup	294	24
Beans, Pinto (Dry)		Cup	150	10
Broccoli, Fresh	1	Cup	24	3

Protein Source	Serving Size		Calories	Grams Protein
Chickpeas / Garbanzo Beans		Cup	170	10
Kidney Beans (Dry)		Cup	160	11
Lentil (Cooked)	0.5	Cup	115	9
Milk (2%)	8	Oz	140	10
Milk (1%)	8	Oz	110	9
Milk, Skim	8	Oz	86	8
Soybeans (Boiled)	0.5	Cup	127	11
Soy Milk (Tris)	1	Cup	90	3
Soy Milk (Sylvia)	1	Cup	100	6
Wheat Germ	2	Tblsp	50	4
Yogurt, Fat Free	8	Oz	110	11
Yogurt, Nonfat, Lite	8	Oz	90	8
Yogurt, Fat Free, Lite	6	Oz	90	6
Yogurt, Yoplait Original/99% Fat Free	6	Oz	180	6

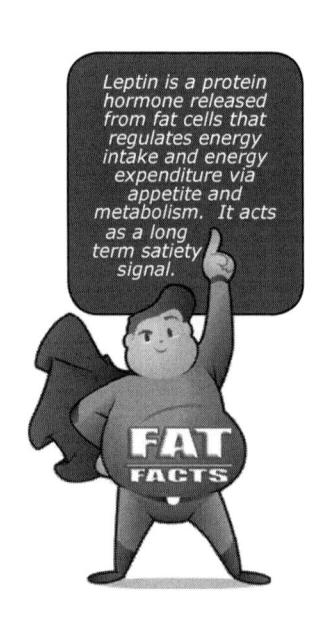

Leptin is a protein hormone released from fat cells that regulates energy intake and energy expenditure via appetite and metabolism. It acts as a long term satiety signal.

FAT FACTS

9

Subtle Ways To Control Calories

Up to this point, I have explained a number of things, including what happens to you when you diet, rapid weight loss techniques, all caloric dependent, to the different macronutrients' importance in long term weight loss maintenance. We have also reviewed some simple principles to help you understand how to modify your calories as you attain and then maintain your goal weight in The Willey Principle and direct ways to control caloric loads. Now we are going to get right to the heart of the matter: Long term maintenance of weight loss by subtle caloric control. The Z Diet consists of, and is simply a detailed way to help you do just that. Every method I am about to review helps control your calories in one form or another. This is a way of life. What I hope to accomplish with this is to teach you **how** to eat, not *what* to eat. There are plenty of good books on what to eat. In my world view, due to economic constraints, preferences and the heartfelt desire to see people maintain their weight loss, I would rather let them eat what they want but at the same time learn how to eat it. This is the concept of the Z Diet. I do not criminalize food, as this causes nothing but stress and failure in the long run. Obviously, some foods are better choices than others, as has been reiterated. As you have heard me say a few times by now, I do not believe there is such thing as a bad food, just bad eating plans.

The nine steps I am about to cover I have been using for years to help people indirectly control their total caloric intake. Obviously, and as mentioned before – a food scale and anal retentiveness are your best bet, but I am more pragmatic than that. There is also some neat research in each of these, in the sense that we know they work for more reasons than just controlling calories. Some act to wake up the metabolism, some help control hunger and others help regulate and balance important brain and gut hormones involved in the whole weight loss, weight gain thing. I will briefly cover a few of these under each heading. This is the meat of the Z Diet. This is a simple way expressing how to eat for long term weight loss maintenance.

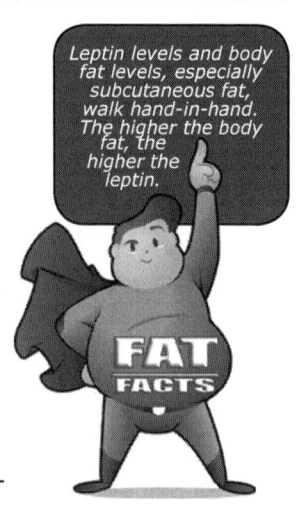

Leptin levels and body fat levels, especially subcutaneous fat, walk hand-in-hand. The higher the body fat, the higher the leptin.

Biggest meal in AM, smallest in PM

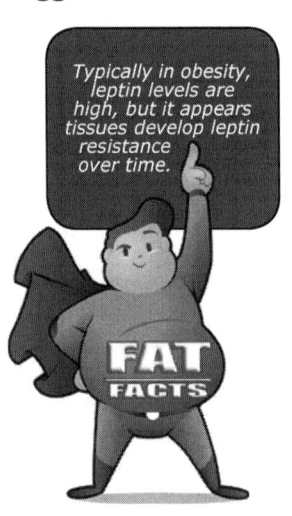

Typically in obesity, leptin levels are high, but it appears tissues develop leptin resistance over time.

We have all heard the old adage: Eat breakfast like a king, lunch like a prince and diner like a pauper. There is a lot of wisdom in this. Of course, a number of studies will tell you that the time a day you eat does not matter, just your total caloric load. I would agree with the fact that total caloric consumption is of enormous value in long term weight loss management. However, I think eating when you first wake up is also of prime importance. As always, I will keep it brief with a mention of just a few studies that point to its importance. As for people that work swing shifts or night shifts, I will use the term 'breakfast' interchangeable with the 'meal you eat when you first get out of bed', no matter what time that is.

I like to discuss real life analogies with my patients; the one concerning the importance of breakfast involves the Indianapolis 500. As obvious as it may sound, the correlation is direct for any engine i.e. your body and a multi-million dollar race car. Not one of the drivers in that well known race starts the race on a half tank of gas. Nor do they start the race without checking the oil pressure or their tires. Yet, it is a common thing to hear in my weight loss practice the 'I don't eat breakfast because...' and it continues to amaze me. No matter what your excuse may be, breakfast is an essential part of long term weight loss.

> Low leptin levels cause hyperphagia (lots of eating), reduced thermogenesis, and a fall in reproductive hormones, thyroid hormones, and immune function.

From the National Weight Control Registry we learn that there are four behavior characteristics of people who have achieved long term weight loss including: eating a low-fat diet, eating breakfast almost every day, frequent self-monitoring of weight, and participation in a high level of physical activity. We have covered direct ways to control calories in the last chapter, one of them being to eat a lower fat diet. Numbers three and four above will be covered shortly.

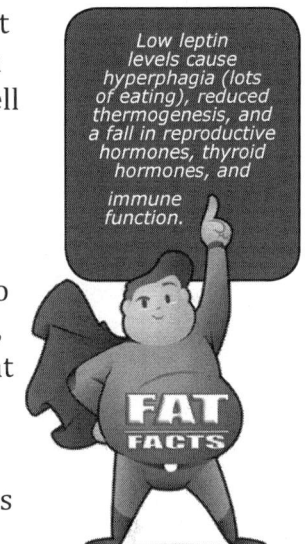

Eating a good sized first meal does seem to be a tool in the long term weight loss paradigm. We cannot say exactly why, but a few theories indicate that insulin sensitivity is highest when you first wake up, and therefore calories you consume are better utilized. There is some research that points out that in free living adults, skipping breakfast was/is associated with a higher degree of obesity (1). An excellent paper by a gentleman named Castro pointed out that eating in the morning increased satiety (the feeling of contentment with your food) throughout the whole day and that eating breakfast lowers the total amount of calories you consume throughout the day (2). It has also been shown to have an impact on kids: adolescents in this study showed a coloration between weighing less and eating breakfast (3). I could go on and on, but again, in my attempt to keep this simple and to the point, it simply sums it up to say: eat breakfast.

In my clinical weight loss setting we see a positive benefit of eating breakfast. It is so correlated with long term weight loss maintenance; it is one of the first things we teach in my practice. The primary hesitancies I run into when I mention it are threefold: 1. I do not have time; and, 2. when I do eat breakfast I am hungry all day; 3. I have

Insulin The Wrong Way • How Most People Eat

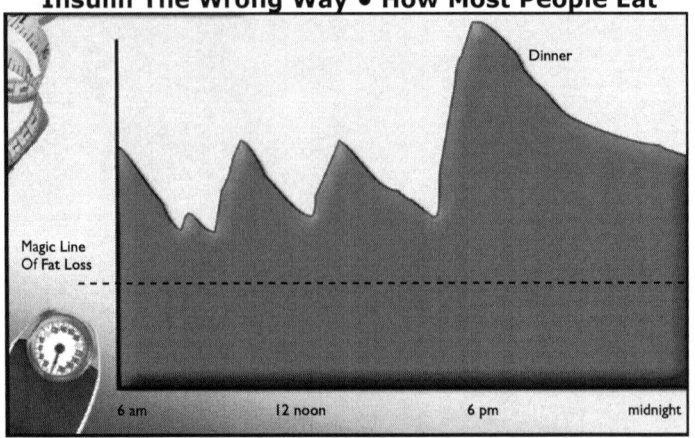

(Graph showing insulin levels throughout the day with Dinner peak, Magic Line Of Fat Loss, from 6am to midnight)

What Insulin Should Be Doing

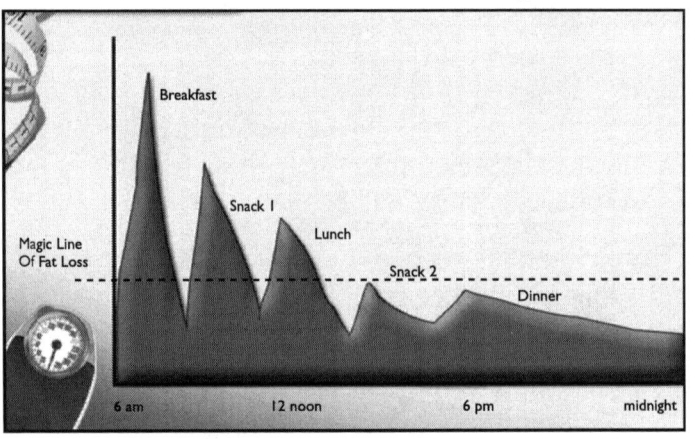

(Graph showing Breakfast, Snack 1, Lunch, Snack 2, Dinner peaks with Magic Line Of Fat Loss, from 6am to midnight)

Insulin The Right Way

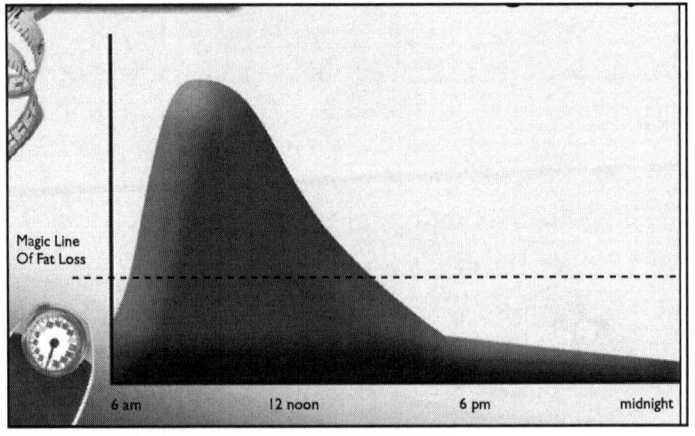

(Graph showing single large peak with Magic Line Of Fat Loss, from 6am to midnight)

never eaten in the morning (because it makes me nauseous, I am not hungry, and a plethora of other excuses), so don't expect me to start now. Let me address all of these:

When I hear people tell me they do not have time, they are being honest. By the time we wake up, get ready for the day, get the kids out the door, and drop the dog off at the vet's - all before heading to work – many of us likely do not have time to eat breakfast. But as I talk about in my book ***What Does Your Doctor Look Like Naked?*** how much time do you have for disease? How badly do you want to lose weight or maintain the weight loss you have already achieved?

Eating a meal when you first wake up takes planning, but it is not impossible. Based on the food timing model I am about to share with you, some of the quick to grab breakfasts (as long as there is adequate protein) are a viable option. At the risk of getting shot: even a fast food option would be ok. In a study published in 2007 under very well controlled conditions a fast food meal was compared to an organic turkey and organic beef meal – the findings: almost every measure of body response to the foods (glucose, insulin, free fatty acids, triglycerides, LDL cholesterol, HDL cholesterol, leptin and ghrelin) measured every 30 minutes for six hours after ingestion were the same. The only one that had a slight change was LDL in the organic beef meal, which showed a decrease (12). Banish the thought, but fast food may be legitimate in this situation, just keep in mind the caloric density of fast food. It is likely to contain a lot more calories than food you prepare at home. Keep in mind, this was one meal. Eating breakfast (or dinner) away from home on a regular basis has been shown to increase weight (1). The simple fact is you need to plan ahead. See below for more detail on planning.

As for the excuse of being hungry all day following breakfast, a number of studies have shown an actually decrease the total number of calories consumed throughout the day. I am most certainly not questioning the hunger, but there is likely a solution to it such as eating more often throughout the day (see below), ensuring adequate protein in your diet, especially breakfast, etc. I encourage people who have this fear to really look at what they eat when they experience the hunger after an AM meal. The majority of the time it is processed, high glycemic cereal, bread, or sugar with zero to none on the protein, so of course they are hungry after breakfast...

As far as the third excuse I hear the 'I have never eaten breakfast because...' I would encourage you to start low and go slow. If you're nauseated by breakfast, find something like a mild fruit with some dairy to start. Starting slowly really works! I have heard it a thousand times over in my clinic. Of all the excuses I hear for not eating breakfast, a number of them come back to the fact; you ate too much before bed, which brings us to our next subtlety in calorie control:

Don't eat before bed

There are plenty of viewpoints that are quick to point out that it does not matter what time of day you eat, it's the total amount of calories you consume that matter. With a bird's eye view of weight loss and particularly long term weight loss, again, I would agree. But this is a chapter on subtle ways to control total caloric intake. Eating right before bed has some consequences and it seems to me when I ask people how they feel going to bed on a full stomach (with the reflux, the nightmares, the indigestion) it becomes intuitive.

Let me tell you from a practical and clinical perspective how powerful avoiding food at night can be. In patient upon patient interview on both the success and failure of dieting, night time food consumption comes up. In real life, night time eating adds up to weight gain and the malfunction of long term weight loss maintenance. Think about it – when does night time eating come in to play? Usually while sitting in front of the boob tube snacking without any conscious thought of what or how much is passing your lips! The calories add up because by bed time your brain is numb to any conscious thought of your waist. Not only that, but if our goal is to get up in the morning and eat breakfast that is not likely to happen if your satiety center is perfectly happy from the night before! I hear all the time "Doc, I am never hungry in the morning, so breakfast is most certainly out of the question". My response, with a universal reply is "how much do you eat before bed?" The answer, always initiated with a nice pause... "a lot" about sums it up. Not only that, but night time food usually consists of the caloric dense sugar or fat filled foods – another sneaky way to increase your total caloric load without thought. Studies back this, as the study I referred to earlier, shows a direct increase in total caloric consumption with late night eating (2)! I have read studies that purposefully place people in a low sugar state at night time (hypoglycemia) causing an increase in first morning hunger and therefore eating, but there are so many variables involved with studies like this, I will not list any as references. I think it does give indication that eating before bed decreases first thing in the morning eating.

Night time eating has been proven to be detrimental to those with gastroesophageal reflux disease (GERD) and asthma. Both conditions are exacerbated with food before bed. Honestly, as a primary care doctor, I very rarely meet a person with a weight problem who does not have one or the other! The simple fact is this: you can assist your total caloric load in an average day by not eating at night. People in my clinic who take this to heart not only lose weight, but use this little suggestion to keep it off! Not eating before bed is an essential part of the Z Diet!

Meal Frequency

I have been a solid proponent of more frequent feeds for a number of years, but not for the common reasons. Almost all of the major diet plans out there suggest at least five meals a day, primarily based on the assumed truth that it would keep your metabolism fired up, and allow you to burn more fat. This originally comes from a study done in the early 1960's by Fabry et al that showed an inverse association between meal frequency and body weight. One theory behind it was based on the Thermic Effect of Food (TEF) I will cover in a minute. Eat more frequently, and you burn more calories because your TEF goes up with the more frequent meals. Since that time, a number of other studies have *not* shown an association between meal frequency and total energy expenditure. Studies evaluating the effect of increased meal frequency on total caloric intake have been inconclusive. What this means is that eating more often does not really change your metabolism. It can change some things metabolically, which is an easy confusion to make between metabolism and metabolic function – they sound the same, but their means are quite different. Things such as postprandial thermogenesis (the heat you produce after eating) and insulin levels (the total peak and a relevant factor we in healthcare use called Insulin's Area Under the Curve) show improvement with more frequent feedings. Lipid or cholesterol profiles also improve with more frequent feedings which may have some great indications for heart related issues (4). The simple fact, however, that eating more often causes weight loss is a misinterpretation of the data. I could also argue that eating more frequently causes weight gain in some, as in their attempt to eat five or six meals a day, some people *increase* the total calories for the day due to food choices and the plain fact of trying to get that many meals down their throat.

You are likely asking by now, why is meal frequency listed as part of the Z Diet? The number of times you eat is important if you are metabolically challenged, as was indirectly mentioned above when I talked about the peaks of insulin being lessened and the area under the curve with insulin response per meal is/are improved. Any improvements with insulin's response to things that cross your lips are important. Therefore, for the metabolically challenged, I encourage it.

From direct observation in my clinic, *eating patterns*, such as meal frequency, have more to do with weight loss, because of the indirect influence on calories. I think this is why early observational studies assumed an increase in metabolism, which there is not, with more frequent feedings. They simply concluded that eating more frequently caused weight loss, due to an increase in metabolism/energy usage.

Eating patterns would include how often you eat, what time of day you eat, etc. For example: in some, eating more frequently helps to control calories if they have tendencies to not eat all day then go all out at night in a full fledge bender. In this case, you would likely do better eating smaller more frequent meals to help curb your evening hunger, particularly when you add protein to each meal for its satiety effects. This is a case of eating less food and therefore indirect caloric control, an essential part of long term weight loss maintenance. This is yet another opportunity to mention the fact that the Z Diet is nothing more than a way to eat.

Meal frequency is also important and a subtle way to control calories if you eat according to your schedule. By this I mean if your schedule allows you three meals a day, eat three meals a day. If your schedule allows for five meals a day, eat five. If you normally get five meals in, but have a rough day and only get three in, so be it. Don't beat yourself up over the number of times you eat a day. I have seen people toss all dietary efforts out the window simply because they could not "eat that often". That is ridiculous. I have had as many clients do well on three meals a day as those who have done well on five meals a day. It comes down to the a simple fact you need to know about yourself; are you the type who eats less throughout the day by eating more frequently? Or are you the type who eats less throughout the day by not eating as frequently? Pick the one where you eat less and live by it. It will be vital to your goal of long term weight loss maintenance.

Majority of carbs early

For those of you who have read any of my other books, you will recognize this section as a rewording of something I call **Food Timing**. I have reworded it for the intended audience of this book, as well as to provide a little more science and view point on this, what I believe is an important topic. The technique of applying food timing to your day simply involves eating the majority of your carbohydrates earlier in the day, and cutting the high insulin stimulating ones i.e. active carbohydrates by late afternoon. This most certainly is a subtle way to keep calories down (hence being in this section of the book) as the majority of us tend to eat big, carb- crammed dinners. But there is more to it. Before I get into the description of Food Timing, please allow me to provide some information I think many of you will find very interesting and directly related to food timing. A topic I call *ChronoNutrakinetics*.

> **FAT FACTS**
> Women have two to three times more leptin than men at any given body fat. It may be one of the reasons men respond so well (and quickly) to diet and exercise compared to gals. As a matter of fact, men below 10% body fat have almost no detectable leptin levels.

When I first started writing diets years ago, I did the classic cut your calories to nothing, make you exercise like crazy, and when it did not work – it was your fault! During medical school, learning about pharmacology and drugs, it occurred to me that food, though not defined as a drug in the strict definition, sure acted like one in my clients bodies (and mine). I started to look at food as a drug, and some amazing things happened. It allowed me to decriminalize a lot of good foods. It allowed me to focus more on the *how to* eat vs. *what to* eat. It also allowed me to develop the food timing model I have written about before. *Chrono**nutra**kinetics* is an extension of that theory, and part of the basis for the theory. To understand it, once again I take you to medical school 101: Pharmacology.

Drugs can be defined as any substance that affects the process of living. *Pharmacology* is the study of drugs. The branch of pharmacology that studies the fate of drugs in the body, as to their absorption, distribution, metabolism, and elimination is called *pharmacokinetics*. In slightly simpler terms, it is the study of *what the body does with the drugs* ingested. *Pharmacodynamics* is the study of the biochemical and physiological affects of drugs and their mechanisms of action, i.e. *what the drug does to the body*.

Chrono**pharma**cokinetics (chrono = time, pharma= drugs, kinetics = having to do with change) is the time-dependent changes in kinetics, which may proceed from circadian variations at each step, e.g. absorption, distribution, metabolism and excretion of drugs or foods in a system. In other words, a particular drug's effectiveness or side effect may be more observable based on when it was taken. The amount of the drug, what the drug was taken with, etc. all come into play - but so does the time of day you ingest the drug, based on our natural daily cycles (sleep/wake, etc.)

When someone reports to my office with a bacterial infection, my choice of treatment, or anti-bacterial in this instance, is based on a huge set of variables. What bug am I trying to kill? What are the side effects of this drug? Does the patient have problems or allergies to this type of drug? What are some of the interactions this drug could have with other drugs, herbals, supplements, and food? How many milligrams would be appropriate for this patient's weight? How many times a day does this patient need to take this drug to achieve adequate effect? For how long? The list goes on...

We in the medical field have yet another variable to consider: what time of day would this drug be most appropriate? The answer to this question is based on chronopharmacokinetics. Why is this important? Because we have more and more "once a day drugs" available to prescribe to our patients and we want to optimize drug affects and/or decrease adverse drug reactions (ADRs) by timing medications with regard to biological rhythms (5).

Chronopharmacokinetics, interestingly enough, shows us that the optimal dosing time sometimes is not the time expected from the perspective of pharmacokinetics. Most, if not all of you reading this, have discussed with your doctor using aspirin as a preventative measure for heart attacks, strokes, and colon cancer. Under the guise of pharmacokinetics, we have been taught that the bioavailability of aspirin in the morning is twice as high as in the afternoon, so we suggest our patients take it in the morning. However, recent evidence-based data favor bedtime dosing of low-dose aspirin to decrease side effects and optimize prevention (6-9)!

We have also begun to realize that the way we treat elevated blood pressure or hypertension (HTN) may need some upgrading, particularly in people with resistant hypertension or hard to treat cases. To date, current thought has been to increase dosage of HTN medications or add more medications on board to get the desired result. But within the realms of chronopharmacokinetics, dosing time may be more important for blood pressure control and for the proper modeling of the circadian blood pressure pattern, rather than just changing the drug combination (10). This has profound effects for lowering ones blood pressure and direct implications in the reason for doing so: a decrease in cardiovascular disease.

Another prime example is that of Non-steroidal Anti-inflammatory Drugs or NSAID's. This is a group of medications in the pain relieving, fever reducing anti-inflammatory area such as Ibuprophen®, Indocin, etc. A number of the NSAID drugs have been shown to have fewer side effects when taken at night vs. the day. One article pointed out that taking NSAID's in the morning doubled the gastrointestinal side effects such as ulcers and bleeding (11).

A number of cardiac drugs, anti-depressants, and other medications have also been found to modify or improve outcomes when one takes into account *when* they are taken. The last specific one I will mention here is the thyroid medication Levothyroxine Sodium, as I am more than certain a number of you reading this are either on thyroid medication or have asked your doctor about thyroid medication. Chronopharmacokinetics tells us that taking thyroid medication at night on an empty stomach will improve your TSH or Thyroid Stimulating Hormone test, versus taking it in the morning before breakfast. In other words, the timing of the medication is as important as the medication itself.

I am providing you mind-numbing information for the purpose of case. A lot of the knowledge behind *Food Timing* is based in chronopharmacokinetics and therefore chrononutrakinetics as I will now describe. The great part about food timing is it makes sense, both from a scientific stand point and, more important, in the area of weight loss, an achievable stand point. *The Z Diet teaches you how to eat.*

So if we look at food as a drug, it would have drug like properties and actions – ask anyone what they do when they are depressed or down – five bucks says they have a favorite drug (food) they turn to. Knowing this, we know food must have some hormonal actions and variations that would make it very much drug like.

Most of the thinking over the last twenty or so years on our obesity epidemic, disease problems, and their direct relationship to one another has been in the area of pharmacodynamics as defined above. In other words, all the focus has been on what food does to the body. The blame has been placed on the food. In this light, it is easy to make one food a criminal, while exalting another. The Z Diet and food timing focuses on the pharmacokinetics of food. In other words, what the *body does with the foods* ingested. From this conjecture we delve into chrono***nutra***kinetics.

Chrono***nutra***kinetics has to do with *when* you eat your food must be as important as *what* you eat and how much you eat. A simple example is the rise of Insulin with the intake of carbohydrates. Using The Z Diet terminology, the zeitgeber is carbohydrates and the internal response is the elevation of insulin, and all of its consequences including the programming of your internal clock to crave carbohydrates at certain times of the day, eat before you go to bed, etc. Did you ever stop to think why you always crave sugar in the late afternoon or before bed? I will tell you why: you programmed your internal clock to do so according to what you had to eat (your zeitgeber) earlier that day and possibly the day before. That is why following The Z Diet plan works so well for long term weight loss. When you take into account all of the factors or steps involved with The Z Diet, you start to change your internal response to food. You reset your clock to a more appropriate schedule and thereby start to benefit from food and not get damaged by it. That is the concept behind *food timing*.

It is extremely important for every imaginable health initiative (weight loss, muscle gain, lowering cholesterol, controlling and/or preventing diabetes, decreasing osteoarthritis, etc.) to know *when* to utilize the foods we like to eat. The timing of food intake in relation to our sleep/wake cycle, exercise, work, playtime, and all the other activities of daily living is what needs to be understood. Once this has been embedded, you will begin to see results of your quest for all the above mentioned health proposals on a new level. You will actually learn to profit from foods that, under the pharmacodynamics theory, would be considered horrifying and still be equipped to maintain your long term weight loss.

The research in this area is exorbitant especially if you look at the sports literature and the relation of nutrient intake to sports timing, particularly in the area of recovery and muscle building. I discuss that in some detail in **Better Than Steroids** so I will not repeat it in The Z Diet. I would encourage you to read that book if you are interested in the topic, the Pre- and Post-workout meal chapters in particular, as their applications can be translated beyond the world of bodybuilding.

The implications are enormous for the concept of food timing. I first described the importance of it in the 1990's in a few of my articles and put to use with all of my clients. Since that time no studies have been done that precisely prove or disprove food timing (there are a few in progress as I type this sentence, however). The research that points to food timing is gargantuan! This can all be gathered together to demonstrate how effective food timing is and will be for you on The Z Diet.

Previously, we discussed insulin and its actions and how that can be translated into optimal health and weight loss. Relative to that discussion is insulin's involvement in building tissue, particularly lean tissue and fat tissue. Insulin is responsible for the storage of energy in both fat and muscle. It deposits this energy into either fat or muscle based on food timing, activity level, when we ate last, the last time insulin was raised (in response to blood sugar) and a variety of other factors. Again, avoiding the esoteric, using insulin's response to food, we will develop a timing system to optimize fat loss and maintain or gain lean mass.

Generally speaking, the body will not utilize fat when sugar is present to burn and use for energy. We are survivalists, and our bodies will do anything to protect that fat for what they believe to be the up and coming starvation they will be required to endure. If we repeatedly feed them active carbohydrates throughout the day, we cause insulin to continually spike, thereby setting up the environment for fat storage. Energy in the form of active carbohydrates is present to feed the brain and the body is as happy as can be. It is never required to turn to fat stores for energy.

What we want to do is tell the system we need to burn fat for energy. How? We have to decrease the amount of sugar present, thereby decreasing the insulin and forcing the body to turn to fat stores. This is, of course, a gross oversimplification, but it makes the point. Make your body burn fat by decreasing the active carbohydrates throughout the day.

In an ideal situation, we utilize active carbohydrates at two times during the day. The first is first thing in your morning upon waking from our overnight "fast". The second is immediately after a workout (if applicable). This is because exercise utilizes the storage form of sugar in the muscles, and sets up the environment for needing to replenish energy. This causes insulin to rise and deposit the energy into our now hungry muscles. Optimally, one would get up and exercise, *then* eat active carbohydrates, as this would combine the best of both worlds in the quest for long term weight loss maintenance. The rest of the day, we slowly decrease our active carbohydrates, allowing a drop in sugar and resulting in a drop in insulin. Our body is then forced into fat burning mode, because insulin is no longer depositing sugar.

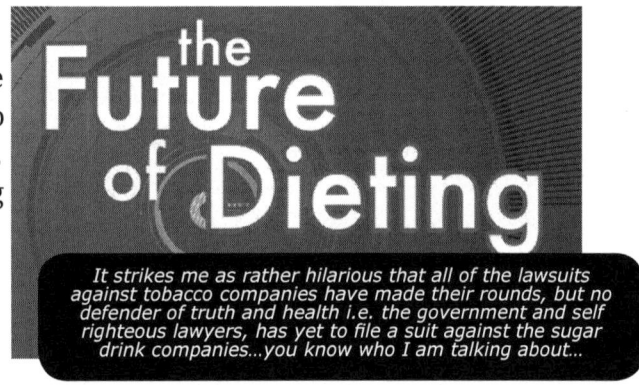

> the Future of Dieting
>
> It strikes me as rather hilarious that all of the lawsuits against tobacco companies have made their rounds, but no defender of truth and health i.e. the government and self righteous lawyers, has yet to file a suit against the sugar drink companies...you know who I am talking about...

Let's review how we can use this tid-bit of the Z Diet to maintain long term weight loss: The Z Diet professes what is ideal physiologically: We go to bed on an empty stomach and wake up in the morning after our overnight fast with insulin sensitivity is at its highest. We then have our biggest active carbohydrate meal of the day, spike insulin, and store that energy in the muscles for growth and maintenance of our lean mass tissue. We ensure adequate protein is available at every meal, eat according to our schedules throughout the day, and slowly decrease our active carbohydrate intake, allowing a steady drop in insulin, causing the body to return to fat stores for energy while we are carrying out our daily activities. This, too, as I have mentioned is a subtle way to decrease your total calories taken in throughout the day. The Z Diet in a nut- shell.

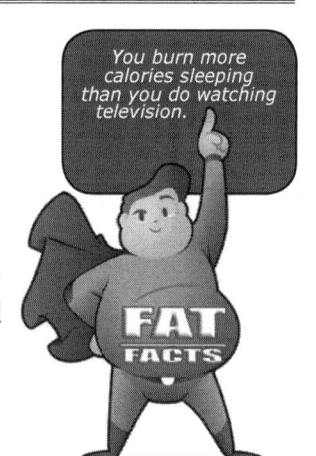

> You burn more calories sleeping than you do watching television.

FAT FACTS

I have seen food timing work over and over in my clinical practice without any other variables. I admittedly hate using testimonials, as everyone has a price and can be asked to say whatever you want them to, but I can provide you with some case studies: a couple of patients whose medical charts document the benefits of food timing or simply eating the majority of their carbohydrates early. Actually, I have dozens of them but as I am a middle of the road person, let me give you a couple of middle of the road examples i.e. not too extraordinary, but at the same time substantial weight loss with nothing more than cutting carbs in the evening. The first is a fellow doctor in my town. He had heard of a few of my theories on weight loss, so he and his wife started having lean meats and vegetables at night, removing the traditional carbohydrates he grew up with – his results: he lost fifteen pounds in four weeks, and admittedly did *nothing* else. The other example I will give is a bit broader. In my practice I give everyone a personalized eating plan with menus, shopping lists – the works. I visited with a 47 year old gentleman exactly two months before he came back in for follow up. Before I went in the room, my assistants did his weight and body composition. In short, he had lost 20+ pounds and put on lean mass. As I happily went into the room to give him the traditional high five for such success, I assumed the menus were the secret to his triumph. He was quick to inform me "Doc, I never used them! I simply did what you said when we first met: started eating breakfast, ate according to my schedule, cut carbohydrates out by mid afternoon, and did not eat right before bed! That is all I did, and I have never felt better!"

Eating the majority of your carbohydrates early is a powerful technique in long term weight loss maintenance. As a subtle way to control calories, and all of the other mechanisms at work – I highly suggest it become a part of your long term weight loss accomplishment!

Energy OUT

Energy out is a way to describe the use of calories. The easiest and most effective solution to durable weight loss is keeping the number of calories you burn up every day. This is most effectively accomplished with a good, daily exercise routine. This subheading was actually titled Exercise originally, but I think it is important for your long term weight loss maintenance goals to understand all the components of your total daily energy expenditure.

There are four primary components of total daily energy expenditure: Resting Energy Expenditure (REE), The Thermic Effect of Exercise (TEE), the Thermic Effect of Food (TEF), and Non-Exercise Activity Thermogenesis (NEAT) and included in that, Spontaneous Physical Activity (SPA).

Resting Energy Expenditure (REE) is the amount of calories or energy your body is utilizing to keep you alive. It provides the fuel for your heart to beat, your brain to function, your liver to process chemical reactions, etc. It comprises the greatest amount of energy use, estimated at around 60 to 70 percent of your total daily energy usage. The REE is somewhat of a set thing. It increases as your size increases, (contrary to popular belief, most large people's metabolisms are actually higher than those of people of smaller size), tends to change a little based on your general activity level, and can be modified to some extent with the amount of muscle you have. Some people, as we are all aware, just have faster metabolisms (REE's) and tend to get away with a lot more than some of the rest of us. We can thank or curse genetics for that one.

The Thermic Effect of Exercise (TEE) is the energy or calories you use while doing specific, *planned*, movement to purposefully burn calories. Some authors will classify your job activity under this heading, stating that a construction worker has a much greater TEE than a secretary. However, I have found a better common sense application working with patients to place your job under the final category NEAT.

TEE is the amount of calories you burn while performing exercise - planned, purposeful exercise such as going to the gym, going for a run or a bike ride. This is important to differentiate from NEAT and SPA activity, because I (and most diet writers) include it in your daily caloric calculations/amounts. In applying TEE to the Z Diet and the quest for long term weight loss maintenance, exercise more, increase your portion sizes, stay weight neutral. Exercise less, decrease your portion sizes, and stay weight neutral. I tell each and every one of my patients that exercise is not beneficial for weight loss per say, but it is vital for weight loss maintenance. Let me get into that just a little deeper for your understanding:

Exercise seems to be a thorn in many a shoe when it is the *only* lifestyle change for people attempting to lose weight. Your calories out or energy expenditure can never match the calories you put in your mouth, unless you go from zero miles per hour to 5 miles per hour and do not change your eating, you may have an initial drop in weight. On the same note, if you go from 10 miles an hour to 50, you may notice a drop in weight as well – truly a function of calories in to calories out. The problem arises as that weight tends to plateau off much more quickly than we hoped or expected. The reason? For the sake of our argument the answer is twofold. The amount of calories we tend to eat and the body's amazing ability to adjust to what we are doing.

Look at the Table at the end of this chapter. It shows the calories spent doing one solid hour of activity, based on weight. This would demonstrate that a 155 pound person walking 3.5 mph, uphill no less for one hour would burn a mere 422 calories (that is equivalent to a small Cold Stone Creamery dessert Ice Cream Cheesecake). I included this table to show that the number of calories you burn with exercise usually comes nowhere close to the calories you put in your mouth.

And a quick little side note here - If you walked on a treadmill at the gym, pay no attention to the calories that lying piece of equipment says you have burned. Too many variables are involved in caloric usage computation – it's wrong and most likely on the overestimated side! Unless you cut back on what goes into your mouth, attainable weight loss is very hard to do with just exercise. Real life eating vs. exercise examples includes the following:

- If you are a 130 lb person and eat a Big Mac, you have to do 4 hours of walking to break even.

- If you are a 155 lb person and have one Jamba Juice® original, you have to walk for 1 hour and 30 minutes at 3.5 mph uphill to burn up the calories.

- If you are a 155 lb person and have one doughnut, you would have to lift weights continuously, nonstop, for 3 hours to burn it off!

> **FAT FACTS**
> Want to know if the food you are about to eat is quality food (excluding the obvious such as hard candies)? Take you food and run it under your kitchen faucet for 10 seconds. If it survives completely intact, eat it! If it starts to get mangled, throw it away!

Studies have even been done showing this. Miller et al (17) reviewed 493 studies between 1969 and 1994 and compared diet (224 studies), aerobic exercise (76 studies) or diet plus exercise (119 studies) for weight loss in healthy individuals. Diet alone (-10.7 kg) and diet plus exercise (-11 kg) were superior to exercise alone (-2.9 kg) in reducing weight.

This is because it is difficult to match the calories you put into your mouth and you burn on the treadmill. The second reason has to do with our bodies' incredible ability to adjust to what we are doing. With the introduction of exercise into a daily regimen, calories are utilized (as we hoped and wished). You are bound to gain weight with more calories being consumed than utilized, and you will lose weight when caloric expenditure exceeds intake – i.e. the purpose of our gym membership. Unfortunately, our bodies quickly figure this out and subconsciously (or not) start to consume more calories to make up the difference. Homeostasis is one of nature's durable laws – like taxes, it is unavoidable. In reality, the more you exercise, the more you tend to eat. Unless your caloric intake is adjusted (i.e. you work on your diet) your weight loss goals will, yet again, be forfeited.

I will emphasize for likely the third time in the last two pages – exercise is vital to weight loss success, particularly long term weight loss success! You just have to add it to part of the big picture. That is why it is a part of the Z Diet, but only one variable in the grand scheme of things.

The Thermic Effect of Food (TEF) or food tax is the number of calories used to process the food you just ate. In other words, it takes energy to break down, digest, and process food. From the energy to chew it, to the energy to place it in its elemental forms (amino acids from proteins, sugars from carbohydrates, etc.) as well as the distribution of said nutrients to the body. Protein is the most 'expensive' nutrient to digest because when you eat good quality protein (as I reviewed in the food concepts chapter) your body takes the amino acids from the steak you just ate and replaces the amino acids in your muscles, an energy costing event. This is just one of the many reasons I encourage high protein intake no matter what type of eating plan you are on, and learn to play/fluctuate your carbohydrates and fats. The TEF as applied to the macronutrients is best understood in terms of calories utilized. In other words; if I gave you 100 calories of carbohydrate to eat, you would use about 5 of those calories to ingest the other 95 calories, giving carbohydrates a 5% food tax or TEF. If I gave you 100 calories of fat to eat, you would use about 3 of those calories to ingest the other 97 calories, giving fat a 3% food tax or TEF. If I gave you 100 calories of protein to eat, you would use about 15-25 of those calories to ingest the other 75-80 calories, giving protein a 15 - 25% food tax or TEF. Applying this information to real life weight loss maintenance; make sure you get your protein in!

Non-Exercise Activity Thermogenesis (NEAT) and Spontaneous Physical Activity (SPA) tends to fall under the same classification mostly for ease. I want to break them down a little and provide an explanation as to why I include your activities of daily living i.e. your job/what you do all day, under NEAT/SPA.

In clinical practice, I try to define to my patients the importance of calories in to calories out. I cannot recall the number of times I have been told "I do not know why I cannot lose weight! I do so much walking at work" or "There is no way my weight came back! I work construction, hard manual labor everyday!" I discuss in a few different places in this book the amazing ability of the body to adapt to given environments and stresses. The homeostatic mechanisms to find a balance far outweigh your ability to utilize calories doing things you do every day. Simply put, and reiterated in other places, if you use 500 calories doing your everyday job, you eat 500 calories to balance it out, hence your inability to lose weight as a busy construction worker. The same applies with weight regain. Recall we discussed both in the introduction and in the chapter on quick weight loss that diets restrict calories in, or make you burn more – there is no other secret to them. Once you go back to normal, and stop your 'diet', this simply means you are no longer restricting calories or burning more calories (most likely with added exercise). So no matter what your job or daily activities are, weight will never be lost, and it will be easily regained (unless you apply the principles of the Z Diet).

NEAT in the big picture is vital in weight loss maintenance. Let's say you exercise 1 hour a day, your TEE calories if you will. NEAT can be defined as the calories being burned the other 23 hours a day. Once thought to be somewhat important, it is now realized to be very important. For those of you paying attention, you just included your sleeping hours in the non-exercising hours of the day. Recall what I mentioned in the blurb on sleep a few chapters ago: no sleep, no weight loss. This is due to the fact that sleep deprivation lowers your Leptin levels and raise your levels of Ghrelin, with a net increase in extremes of hunger. Sleeping burns very few calories, but its net effect on weight control, due to hormonal and recovery reasons, is of absolute necessity. So let's say you exercise 1 hour a day, and sleep for a lovely 8 hours a day. Now NEAT activity is confined to the 15 hours a day leftover. What you do with your body during these 15 hours is vital for your long term weight loss goals.

It would seem, and most certainly apparent to all of you desk jockeys that blame your job for your fatness, that sitting behind a computer screen for the majority of these hours is partially responsible for your weight gain/regain. Your right. Stud-

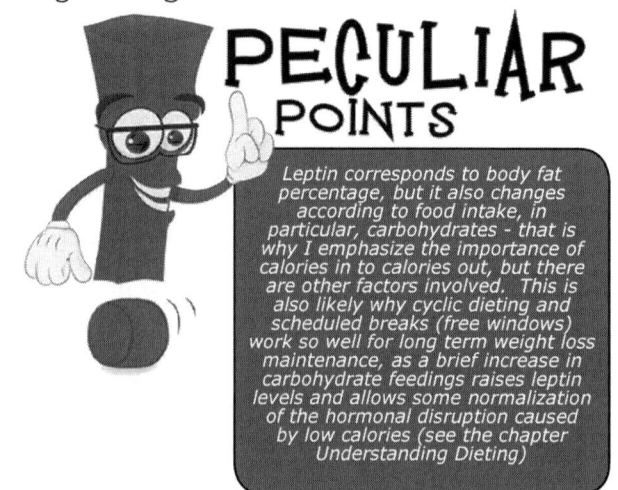

PECULIAR POINTS

Leptin corresponds to body fat percentage, but it also changes according to food intake, in particular, carbohydrates - that is why I emphasize the importance of calories in to calories out, but there are other factors involved. This is also likely why cyclic dieting and scheduled breaks (free windows) work so well for long term weight loss maintenance, as a brief increase in carbohydrate feedings raises leptin levels and allows some normalization of the hormonal disruption caused by low calories (see the chapter Understanding Dieting)

ies have shown that when you are doing anything that involves minimal movement, whilst on your butt, yet still involving your brain to some degree (typing, TV, Facebook®, video games, email, etc.) you set up a situation that drives your mouth to high calorie dense sugar and fat filled foods. This is likely due to the brains utilization of blood sugar while performing these tasks. In other words, staying up all night (sleep deprivation) and playing on the Internet (non-movement, on your butt activity while using your brain), causes a lot of fat gain/re-gain.

> *Insulin plays a hefty role in weight/fat regulation and it seems that women's brains and men's brains differ (go figure) in response to leptin and insulin. Men's brains respond more to insulin and women's respond more to leptin. As a matter of fact, injecting a male rat with estrogen increases its response to leptin.*

Getting up and running around your office every so often at work or while on the computer is a NEAT way to help keep the weight off. It really starts to add up over time

That's how you use NEAT to your benefit with long term weight loss success. Move as often as possible, whenever possible, and watch your eating. This includes parking farther away from your destination, using stairs instead of the elevator – you have heard them all.

SPA, the way I classify it, is the activity of a pickup basketball game, or a brief jog down the street to the bank to deposit a check. SPA activity, like NEAT's caloric amount is not something to include in your weight loss program, but is essential for weight loss maintenance. Just like NEAT activity, get out there and move as often as you can: play tennis, basketball, a pick up football game, wrestle with your kids or spouse – just move!

Cyclic Eating

In my book ***Better Than Steroids***, I spent a lot of time discussing different eating plans and, more important, the benefits of alternating between the different eating plans for the goals of those readers. In the Z Diet, changing types and variety of eating plans is also important for its benefits in long term weight loss maintenance. The ease of monotony can be argued for long term weight loss, and a number of very successful people in this area eat the same thing, day in and day out. In discussing it with them, they are quick to point out that they basically follow the premise of the Z Diet because eating the same foods everyday allows them to consciously and subconsciously control their calories, eat to their schedule, control hunger and urges, and maintain their weight loss. They still apply scheduled breaks, as I will cover shortly, but the simplicity of this style of eating works for them.

Not everyone can do that due to schedule conflicts, travel, type of occupation they are in, and flat out boredom with that kind of eating. That is OK, and this is where cyclic eating can be of great benefit in long term weight loss control. The assertion behind cyclic eating is simple: change what you are doing every so often for the psychological break and the physiologic advantage. This allows subtle caloric control in the big picture of things. It also allows you to alternate different foods and food types in and out of your daily eating plan, and as this can be very advantageous in the long run. From a psychological stand point, it allows a well controlled break while you are still following your long term weight loss plan. From a physiological stand point, it is a mini version of the topic I will be discussing next in scheduled breaks. Recall from **Understanding Dieting** all of the physiologic changes that occur with caloric restriction. The majority of them find a new baseline in most people when they are able to maintain long term weight loss; however, there are those who will constantly battle those changes as their bodies are doing their best to regain some of the weight lost. Cyclic eating, for lack of better words, shocks the system (hormones in particular such as leptin) into continually keeping up with what you are doing and how you are changing your eating.

Cyclic eating involves changing the amounts of carbohydrates or calories in your diet by changing portion sizes or amounts in a planned or systematic fashion. Carbohydrates are the easiest way to change things around, and cycle your eating style. This is done simply by increasing the amount of carbohydrates and their portion sizes for a few days consistently and then going back to your long term amounts. I discussed this in Macronutrient Breakdown as the Modified Carb Drop (MCD). In the big picture, it is important to always keep your protein portions at your baseline suggested amounts of 1 gram per pound of scale weight *the majority of the time.* Increasing protein portions for the short run, while decreasing carbohydrate amounts, is an excellent way to cycle your eating, but never let your protein portions slip too low, too long.

With this method, your total caloric load should remain constant. This is done by substituting your protein portions for carbohydrates and visa versa. It can also be done, and of great benefit to increasing calories for the short run in a controlled fashion (I will cover an uncontrolled increase in calories in the next section). This is done simply by increasing your portion sizes for a few days, and then going back to your regular long term weight loss maintenance amounts.

Both methods can be done in a variety of ways: cycle your eating for a few days in a row i.e. cut back a couple of portions of protein and substitute some carbohydrates in their place, and then increase your protein portions while cutting back on your carbohydrate portions for another few days and repeat it. Find the amounts and timing between high/low carbohydrates that work best for you and your schedule. This style of cyclic eating works very well with things such as work weeks – lower carbohydrates throughout the week while at work and in a controlled scheduled environment and then higher carbohydrates over the weekend when there is less demand on your schedule. Weekends are also the time when you are more likely to go on a date, or out to eat, or to a party – all of which almost universally force higher carbohydrates on you. This allows you to control your eating, rather than your eating controlling you.

Let me provide you with a real life example from one of my patients:

> She is a 45-year-old, 150 pound hormonally challenged female, who has visited her doctor (me!) and found hormone balance. She has lost her excess weight, and found she does very well at roughly 1400 calories a day. She eats 150 grams of protein a day (1 gram of protein per pound of scale weight) and therefore gets 600 calories a day from protein (1 gram of protein has 4 calories. 4 x 150 = 600). She uses her hand to portion foods and on an average day eats a lot of fruit and vegetables, and keeps her active carbohydrates in her diet around breakfast. On average, she eats the same amount of carbohydrates as she does protein, and considers about 200 calories a day as inci-

dental.

Using cyclic eating, she rotates a few weeks of higher protein and lower carbohydrates into her daily plan. She does this by simply decreasing her servings of carbohydrates, and increasing her servings of protein. She follows this by doing just the opposite for a week or so; going back to 150 grams of protein a day and doubling her carbohydrates for awhile.

She then goes back to her basic style of eating, and repeats the process a few weeks later. If you read **Better Than Steroids,** I have simply described a Zig Zag eating plan (both calories and carbs) as well as a controlled, short term glycogen supercompensation or re-feed.

Another simple approach is reapplying the techniques or eating plans you used to get the weight off in the first place, for a short while, then going back to the Z Diet for long term weight loss maintenance.

With short run changes in your eating plan as described, a few things occur, including alternating between anabolic (periods or growth) and catabolic (periods of breakdown) states in the muscle, as well as feeding the brain the occasionally wanted and sought after treat or food item. There has always been an argument as to whether this type of intermittent cyclic eating benefits the metabolism. My guess, as is typical with my down the middle style, is that it does in some and not in others. There is little question as to the metabolic effects of scheduled breaks, which we will cover now.

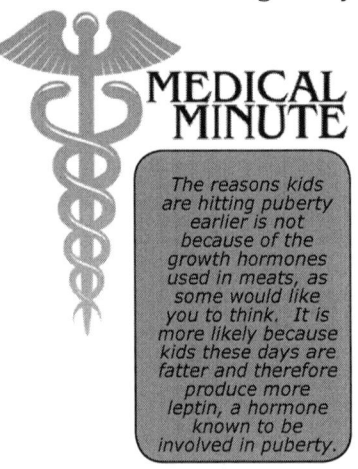

MEDICAL MINUTE

The reasons kids are hitting puberty earlier is not because of the growth hormones used in meats, as some would like you to think. It is more likely because kids these days are fatter and therefore produce more leptin, a hormone known to be involved in puberty.

Scheduled Breaks

I have been a huge proponent of breaks in one's dietary regimen for a number of years. From the seasoned body builder to the veteran dieter, breaks in the dietary regimen are of great benefit. As with cyclic eating, the benefits are both psychological and physiological. When I discuss breaks from your dietary norm, I mean full on overeating, face stuffing with every delectable treat you can think of, which usually comes down to high sugar and fat filled foods and tons of active carbohydrates which, I am most certain, is what you think of too – perfect! We are on the same page…

I discussed short term breaks in **What Does Your Doctor Look Like Naked?** in the chapter entitled **The Free Window**. Those breaks ranged from a single meal or three hour window to a full day or weekend break, intermittently placed in a dieter's grand scheme of things. The difference between what I discussed there and what I will be covering here is time frames and the approach to setting up a scheduled break. **The Free Window** also concerned people who where/are currently in the process of *weight loss*. Scheduled breaks in the Z Diet plan are for people with the goal of *long term weight loss maintenance*.

The approach to setting up a scheduled break is simple, as is the time frame I am going to suggest. The time frame can range anywhere between one and two full weeks, possibly more if you watch your fat and lean mass and how they are responding to the scheduled break. Planning for it is simply looking at your calendar, and *writing down* the weeks you are going to not give a flying hoot about what crosses your lips. This can be done around holidays, your birthday, a vacation – you get the idea. The important thing about setting up your scheduled breaks is *writing them down*, or putting them in your Google® calendar or on your hand held communication device. You have to *schedule* your scheduled break for it to really work. Scheduled breaks in my office are called prescription breaks. I write out, on a prescription pad, an assignment to take a set time frame off all thoughts of me, the diet plan patients are on, and I have them mark it in their calendars right in front of me (when possible).

I will tell you why it is so vital to write down and actually schedule your break: years of doing this has taught me some real life truisms that cannot be avoided. If someone in an all out quest for long term weight loss maintenance puts their best foot forward and really tries to follow their eating plan 24/7, including holidays and vacations and they have a slip up, my experience tells me that they are very unlikely to get back on that band wagon once fallen. Hence, yet another reason for all the yo-yo dieting that goes on. But if someone purposefully *plans* a scheduled break, *writes it down*, and *aims* for it – they have no problem resuming their long term weight loss program after. I have seen it over and over in clinical practice!

There are even a couple of studies that refer to the power of scheduled breaks, one in particular I will mention here. In *Obesity Research*, February 2003 (13), an article discusses two researchers by the name of Wing and Jeffery, who set out to see if people would fall off the wagon when told to take a break from their dietary efforts. The article was titled "*Prescribed breaks as a means to disrupt weight control efforts*". They divided 142 subjects into three groups. One group was instructed to take a long break of six weeks from their dietary efforts; a second group was told to take a short break of 2 weeks intermittently throughout the study; and, a third group acted as the control, i.e. taking no breaks. Each group member received a standard 14 week behavioral weight loss program. The long break group was given a break at week 7 and the short break group was given two week breaks at weeks 3, 6, and 9. The break groups were instructed to stop all dietary efforts during the prescribed breaks.

As a number of studies do, this one did not perform as hoped by the researchers. They set out to develop a method to experimentally produce weight loss relapse; however, they found something very intriguing. Breaks produced a slowing of weight loss and in some cases a slight regain, but neither was clinically significant as compared to the control group. Total weight lost was similar for all three groups at the end of the study. In other words, the group that dieted without breaks had the same results as those who had both short and long term breaks. Most important, they found that *none of the participants had any problem resuming their diets following the breaks!*

Simply put: when you plan and write down a scheduled break from your long term weight loss efforts, not only will you not gain all of your weight back, but you will have a much easier time getting back on the wagon *when you schedule them!*

When I help someone schedule a dietary break, or an all out feed fest, they not only are replenished psychologically, but have done some amazing physiological adaptations as well. Recall all of the horrible things I discussed a few chapters ago that occur with caloric restriction. They all reverse with scheduled mass feedings! That means your testosterone comes back up followed in short order by your mood and sex drive. Thyroid function returns, as do all the benefits of its work. Growth hormone and IGF-1 increase in concert with an increase in insulin. These all help build muscle and produce an overall anabolic state. The stress hormone cortisol decreases as does that hunger hormone ghrelin. Energy states in the cell and overall increase through the roof, and the hormone from the fat cell Leptin also increases. Leptin's increase alone has many beneficial aspects, including some crossover with a few things mentioned above. In other words, the psychological and physiological adaptations to scheduled breaks are essential for long term weight loss maintenance. They are key component to the Z Diet, and something I would highly encourage you to get your calendar out now, and determine when your next scheduled break will occur! If you decide to go longer than 2 weeks, please be sure to track your lean and fat mass closely, and that brings us to the next step in the Z Diet – tracking results.

Tracking Results

A key component to the Z Diet is tracking your results, and being keenly aware of what your body is doing in relation to your activity and your eating. I have been very sensitive to the fact of tracking importance in a clinical setting, as have my clients. As a matter of fact, when I run into one of them I have not seen in awhile, they are quick to mention the need to get measured again, to see where they are and how they are doing. As I mentioned with the National Weight Control Registry, one of the key characteristics of people who have achieved long term weight loss included frequent self-monitoring of weight.

Scale weight is most certainly the easiest way to follow how you are doing and I encourage using it. How often, I will cover shortly, but I want to spend some time helping you see the importance of incorporating a few other tracking measures that will help you in some detail with your long term weight loss management. I encourage everyone to follow both *subjective* and *objective* measures. Subjective measures can be done with a simple journal or following an actual chart like the one I provided in **What Does Your Doctor Look Like Naked?** They are important, as I would most certainly consider how you feel to be as important as how you look! They are also an excellent way to monitor subtle changes, in particular with your cyclic eating, as knowing how you feel on higher carbohydrates and/or calories is essential in the big picture. Objective data is also vital for a long term weight loss program. Taking a picture of yourself and comparing it frequently to others is an excellent and simple way to follow your status. With the advent of computers and digital imaging, you can easily track and compare how you are maintaining.

I am a big fan of body composition testing so I am going to spend some time here reviewing it. Body composition allows you to differentiate fat and fat free mass. Relying on the scale alone is of benefit, but the importance of adequate lean mass cannot be understated.

I am convinced that part of the problem with most people's inability to maintain long term weight loss is the fact that many of them are not necessarily over fat, but under muscled. In light of this, we have been attacking the fat everywhere we turn without much of a dent in the problem. Why? In particular with long term weight loss maintenance, maybe our focus should be adjusted a little. As tracking data is a key component to the Z Diet, any possibility of a better, longer term solution would be attractive. Maybe we should put some effort into following our lean mass, rather than just our fat mass and/or scale weight. The only way to do that is to measure it.

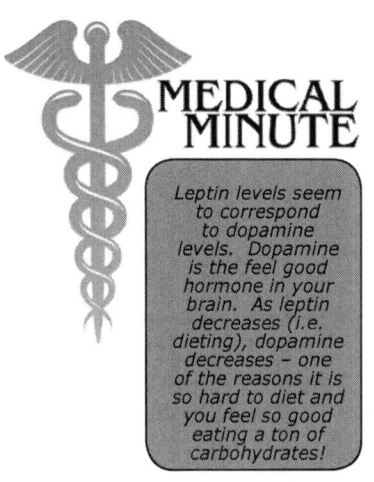

MEDICAL MINUTE

> Leptin levels seem to correspond to dopamine levels. Dopamine is the feel good hormone in your brain. As leptin decreases (i.e. dieting), dopamine decreases – one of the reasons it is so hard to diet and you feel so good eating a ton of carbohydrates!

In my clinic I focus a lot of attention on muscle. How much muscle does this person have, and how much can we build on them using proper diet and exercise techniques? How much are they maintaining on the Z Diet?

As we have discussed, one of the causes of obesity is energy imbalance over a prolonged period of time. Energy in (eating) exceeds energy out (exercise). The alteration of this imbalance can be obtained by varying one or the other. As I mentioned above, the total energy outflow is the sum of resting energy expenditure (REE), the thermic effect of food (TEF), and the energy used related to exercise (TEE). Under most circumstances, REE is the largest component of total energy expenditure (14). Muscle is involved with your REE by the synthesis and break down of muscle protein, so the more muscle you have, the more turnover, the greater number of calories expended.

To give you real numbers: muscle protein synthesis ranges from 0.23 to 0.90 kg/d, once again, dependent on the amount of muscle present. Four mol (short for mole – a unit of amount of substance) of ATP are utilized per mole of amino acids incorporated into protein (15) and the hydrolysis of 1 mol ATP releases 20 kcals of energy (16). This means that the energy released per day as a result of muscle protein synthesis may be as high as 500 kcal/d in a young man with 55 kg of lean mass. I apologize for the science here, but it is important.

Continuing with our real number example, a difference in REE of 500 kcals, based on muscle protein turnover and therefore muscle mass, would lead to a gain or loss of 65 g of fat per day (1 Kg of fat is 7700 kcal). If all things remained constant (no changes in diet or exercise) this would mean that an REE variation of 500 kcal would equate to a gain or loss of 1.95 Kg of fat a month (4.29 lbs). This estimate is actually low, as I have not accounted for the energy expended with the hydrolysis of ATP by way of protein *breakdown*.

This is why I have placed tracking results and specifically measuring body composition under subtle ways to control calories. If you know your lean mass is being maintained on the Z Diet, you have managed to keep your caloric burn elevated! If your lean mass starts to slip, something you can only catch by measuring it, you can take efforts to bring it back up, such as ensuring your quality protein is adequate in your diet, and keeping your body moving with a good exercise program, specifically weight lifting.

Focusing on muscle with body composition testing does three primary things:

1. You focus on metabolism as I mentioned above.
2. Disease prevention. It has been proposed that the metabolic changes of a majority of lifestyle related diseases such as insulin resistance and diabetes occur *before* you get fat, and therefore fat is yet another indicator of inadequate hormonal, cellu-

lar, and biological function. Focusing on muscle prevents that. Another prime example is that of osteoporosis: maintenance of adequate bone density and strength is decidedly dependent on adequate muscle mass and function.

3. Long term success. When you fix your metabolism with proper nutrition and exercise, i.e. you maintain or build muscle, you enable the maintenance of fat loss by, once again, increasing metabolism and maintaining it.

Keeping track of your progress, specifically gains and losses, is an important key to The Z Diet. This area is often overlooked because it seems confusing, too time consuming, or too technical to learn and accurately track. Over the years I have seen both sides. Some people keep impeccable records to track their progress, while others fly by the seat of their once large pants. It always seems to be the case that people who spend the time to learn how to measure and monitor their results, have better and more consistent results than those who do not. Do not overlook the importance of measuring your progress!

Yet one more reason to measure body composition: in my practice I see "skinny-fat" people all the time. Another term used to describe these people is "sarcopenic obesity". Sarcopenia is the supposedly age related decrease in muscle mass with time. This term merely defines a person with a skinny phenotype (how they look), but an atrocious body composition i.e. they are fat! One example of this is the classic over exercisers who, if walking down the street would turn heads with their stealth appearance, but who, if their body composition were measured, would be 40 to 50 percent body fat. I see these people all the time – and they are farther from health than some of my patients who do not have that "look", but who have the body composition we all desire.

There are many ways to measure your body fat, including scales you stand on without shoes on, to hand held devices (bioelectrical impedance) all the way up to a CT scan. Skin fold testing is, I believe, the simplest and best way to measure your body composition. The rational for skin fold testing is that there is a relationship between the fat located in the depots directly beneath the skin and that of internal fat and body density. A special caliper is utilized to measure the skin fold thickness in millimeters at specific sites on the body. The most common sites include the triceps, chest, subscapular area (back), suprailiac (hip region), abdomen, and upper thigh. Skin fold measurements are utilized two ways: The first is to take the sum of all the measurements as a relative degree of 'fat to lean' among individuals. The second way is to use skin folds in conjunction with mathematical equations to predict percentage body fat. These equations are population specific and accurate when similar populations are tested. Advantages to skin fold testing are simplicity, accuracy when done by experienced (or well practiced) persons, and excellence in detecting change when done by the same person, in the same sites, under similar circumstances.

How often you measure your body composition is a question I am asked quite often. That is, like everything to do with dieting, not an easy answer. If you are in the losing stage, fat loss does not occur in a predictable fashion. In other words, some weeks it falls of your body and others it is stuck with super glue. The variables involved with this are tremendous, so let me cover just a couple that will be of importance for utilizing body composition for maintaining your long term weight loss goals. The first is water weight. In the chapter **Quick Weight Loss Approaches**, I cover the water alterations that occur with almost any dietary changes. When you start to diet and measure yourself, you start to lose in a more or less orgasmic linear fashion. Unfortunately, your thrill ends abruptly when the water starts to balance back out, and that once slide like weight loss ends. Even worse, and to use the lovely ladies reading this book as an example, you hit the right time of the month and, even though you have with great furor and gusto stuck to your diet, weight starts coming back on. Water or fat? That's where it gets really tough!

My suggestion is that you pick regular intervals to measure yourself. If you are just starting a weight loss plan (something I am not covering in The Z Diet) you may want to track your body composition a little more often, say once a week, so you can see what water is doing, and how your time of the month or other variables are coming into play. It is also very important to monitor your changes so you can make dietary/exercise changes accordingly, because as I discuss in **Better Than Steroids**, your calorie requirements change with your body composition especially in the weight loss phase.

For those of you reading the Z Diet to help you hold on to your current weight, I believe once a month is ideal to track your body composition and ensure no backsliding is taking place. This is especially true for the young ladies out there who are still menstruating. Follow your body composition once a month, the same time every month. This is about the only way to appreciate water changes, and still be able to follow lean and fat mass. For guys; we still have to be aware of water changes, but not to the same degree as all of those pretty gals. Once or twice a month, under the same conditions is ideal.

If you are interested in utilizing skin fold calipers to track your progress while on The Z Diet, you can find a simple set with an instruction manual at www.eatright4u.com.

When Scheduled, Schedule!

This last life style recommendation does wonders for subtle caloric control. It is a saying I use in my clinic to help people understand the importance of planning ahead. It is another way of reinforcing: **If you fail to plan, Plan to fail.** But it also gives some direction as to how to plan!

Every single one of you reading this book has a schedule. If you are a school teacher or a lawyer, a doctor or a stay at home mom – you have a schedule. Most days of the week, I will use Monday through Friday in my example, you have a set time you wake up, a set time to head off to work or kick the kids out the door. You have a set time to take a break during your busy day, a set time to run the kids to soccer practice or run to the store for little Spencer's school project. We all have schedules the majority of the time.

When Scheduled, Schedule means nothing more than on days you have a set schedule, schedule your food intake! Add thirty minutes to your current schedule and make your food for the day, or at the very least – map it out on your hand held communication device, or iPhone. Know when and where you are going to eat. Know what surroundings you will

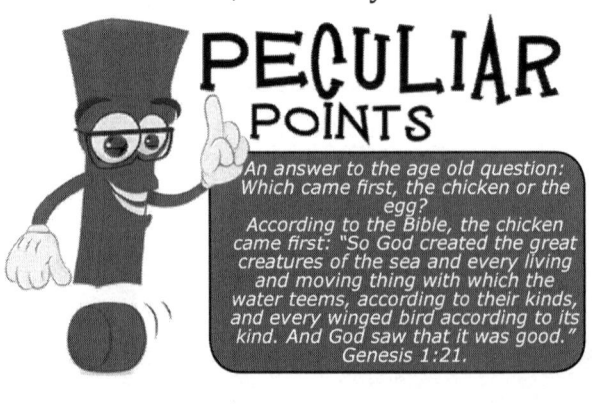

> **PECULIAR POINTS**
> An answer to the age old question: Which came first, the chicken or the egg?
> According to the Bible, the chicken came first: "So God created the great creatures of the sea and every living and moving thing with which the water teems, according to their kinds, and every winged bird according to its kind. And God saw that it was good." Genesis 1:21.

be in for food intake. Will you have a lunch meeting where they serve donuts and cream puffs? If so, you had better plan on bringing your own food or, at the very least, eat before you get there so you are not as tempted. Keeping your food scheduled and planned out on days that are already planned out for you is a great way to subtly control caloric intake. You will control what crosses your lips, not your job, or meeting, nor the traffic jam on the way home – *you* control it, and therefore control your total caloric load for that day.

By the same token: when you are *not* scheduled, be a little more laid back in your food choices. In your quest for long term weight loss maintenance, always look at the big picture. The Z diet, and your ability to keep the weight off, is a *lifestyle* choice. As we are scheduled most days of our lives, planning your food intake on those days will keep you where you want to be, even if you do not do so well on the non-scheduled days. Just as I discussed in Scheduled Breaks, write down your schedule and follow it. Obviously allow for the occasional wrench thrown into your engine, but overall be a high self monitor and plan your food intake on the days life has plans for you.

Summary

In summary, this chapter has covered the nine primary lifestyle steps of the Z Diet and provided you with a powerful tool in your 'keep the weight off' goals. Appling any one of these steps to your life is a great place to start, but taking on all the recommendation of the Z Diet will most certainly help you maintain the weight you have lost. I have also seen these steps help people continue with their weight loss achievements. As an added bonus, whether you are currently in the weight loss arena, giving your best effort with one of the methods I discussed earlier, or considering taking your weight loss further, application of the Z Diet will do nothing but assist you with your goals.

It is important to note that not all of these suggestions work for everyone. That is why it is a lifestyle and I would encourage you to adopt the ones that work for you. For example: Not everyone, for whatever reason, can eat breakfast – so be it! Do not throw the whole concept (in this case book) out the window because you cannot eat breakfast. Use some of the other suggestions that do fit in your new found lifestyle of weight loss maintenance.

In the next chapter we will continue with the Z Diet principles while discussing how to shop and read labels of the food you consume!

ACTIVITY These activities are done for *1* hour, continuously.	CALORIES BURNED		
If you weigh:	130 LBS	155 LBS	190 LBS
Walking, 2.0 mph, slow pace	148	176	216
Walking, 3.0 mph, mod. pace, walking dog	207	246	302
Walking, 3.5 mph, uphill	354	422	518
Running, 5 mph (12 min mile)	472	563	690
Running, 8.6 mph (7 min mile)	679	809	992
Weight lifting, light or moderate effort	177	211	259

1. Ma Y, Bertone ER, Stanek EJ. Association between eating patterns and obesity in a free-living US adult population. Am J of Epiedmiol. 2003; 158 (1). 85-92

2. Castro JM. The time of day of food intake influences overall intake in humans. J Nutr. 2004; 134: 104-111.

3. Albertson AM, Franko DL, Thompson D. Longitudinal patterns of breakfast eating in black and white adolescent girls. Obesity 2007 Sep; 15(9):2282-92.

4. Farshch HRi, Taylor MA, Macdonald IA. Beneficial metabolic effects of regular meal frequency on dietarythermogenesis, insulin sensitivity, and fasting lipid profiles in healthy obese women. Nutr 2005;81:16 –24.

5. Lemmer B, Labrecque G. Chronopharmacology and chronotherapeutics: definitions and concepts. *Chronobiol Int* 1987; 4: 319–29.

6. Markiewicz A, Semenowicz K. Time dependent changes in the pharmacokinetics of aspirin. *Int J Clin Pharmacol Biopharm* 1979; 17: 409–11.

7. Hermida RC, Ayala DE, Calvo C *et al.* Aspirin administered at bedtime, but not on awakening, has an effect on ambulatory blood pressure in hypertensive patients. *J Am Coll Cardiol* 2005; 46: 975–83.

8. Hermida RC, Ayala DE, Calvo C *et al.* Differing administration time-dependent effects of aspirin on blood pressure in dipper and non-dipper hypertensives. *Hypertension* 2005; 46: 1060–8.

9. Kriszbacher I, Koppán M, Bódis J. Aspirin for stroke prevention taken in the evening? *Stroke* 2004; 35: 2760–1.

10. Hermida RC, Ayala DE, Fernández JR *et al.* Chronotherapy improves blood pressure control and reverts the nondipper pattern in patients with resistant hypertension. *Hypertension* 2008; 51: 69–76.

11. Bruguerollea B, Labrecque G. Rhythmic pattern in pain and their chronotherapy. *Adv Drug Dev Rev* 2007; 59: 883–95.

12. Bray GA et al. Hormonal response to a fast-food meal compared with nutritionally comparable meals of different composition. Ann Nutr Metab. 2007 May; 51(2): 163 – 171.

13. Wing, RR. Jeffery, RW. Prescribed breaks as a means to disrupt weight control efforts. Obesity Research. Feb 2003. Vol. 11 No. 2. 287-291

14. Schoeller DA, Ravussin E, Schutz Y, Acheson KJ, Baertschi P, Jequier E. Energy expenditure by doubly-labeled water: validation in humans and proposed calculations. Am J Physiol Endocrinol Metab 1986;250: R823–30.

15. Waterlow JC, Garlick PJ, Millward DJ. Protein turnover in mammalian tissues and in the whole body. Amsterdam, Netherlands: North Holland Publishing Co, 1978:753.

16. Newsholme EA. Substrate cycles: their metabolic, energetic and thermic consequences in man. Biochem Soc Symp 1978;43:183–205.

17. Miller WC et. Al. (1997) A meta-analysis of the past 25 years of weight loss research using diet, exercise or diet plus exercise intervention. Int J Obes Relat Metab Disord 21:941-947

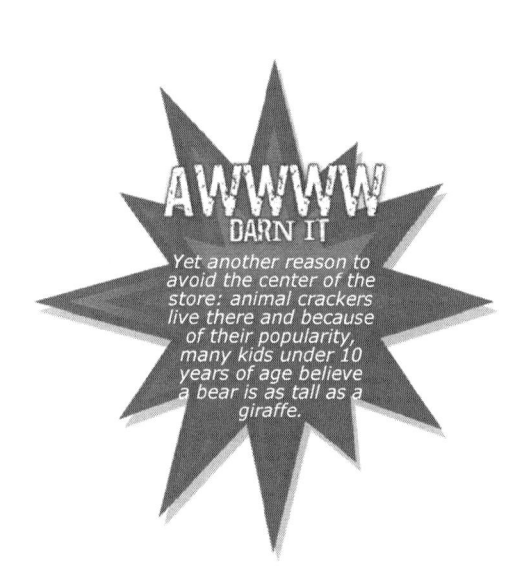

10

How To Shop And Read Labels

As the Z Diet is truly a lifestyle program, one key to the long term solution takes place in a place where most seem to forget how it affects you and your ability to lose weight, much less keep it off: the grocery store. Grocery stores are in the money making business. Yes, they provide a great service, offering all sorts of tastes and textures, necessities and daily needs, but they also are out to make a profit. The way most grocery stores are set up in their actual physical layout suggests this. They are very good at purposefully steering you toward money making goodies, placing certain foods at eye level for the kids, helping you to remember that last minute "need" while in the check out aisle. I am not ripping on them; I am as capitalistic as anyone reading this, and I support them in their efforts to make a buck – that's life. But all of us concerned with long term weight loss maintenance need to be aware of this fact, and I want to provide you with some simple suggestions to ensure you can adhere to the Z Diet and control your weight.

The Layout

Almost every store out there places the items that I would consider good for you and recommended eating while following the Z Diet lifestyle plan, on the periphery. Think about it: mentally walk into your local grocer and take a hard right, walking the outside edge of the store. What you see are the fruits and vegetables, lean meats and dairy, including eggs, milk, fat free yogurt and low calorie cheeses, as well as the frozen vegetables and the frozen lean meats like chicken breasts. This is how I would suggest you shop. Do your shopping on the periphery of the store and avoid the center aisle.

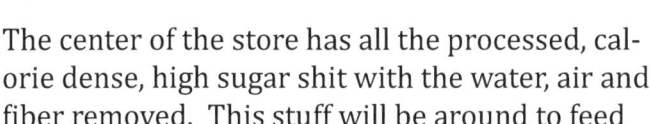

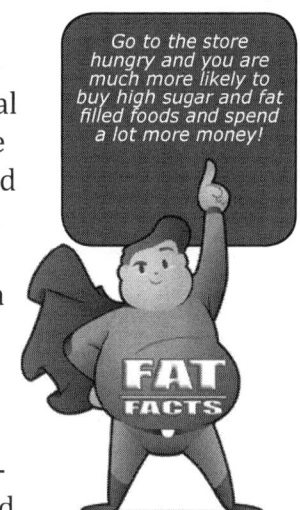

Go to the store hungry and you are much more likely to buy high sugar and fat filled foods and spend a lot more money!

FAT FACTS

The center of the store has all the processed, calorie dense, high sugar shit with the water, air and fiber removed. This stuff will be around to feed the cockroaches after a nuclear bomb hits the area. In general, it is not the best stuff in the world. I am not criminalizing it, nor am I saying you can never traverse the cereal lane for some Lucky Charms®. I am speaking in generalities and the big picture, as you recall.

Buy Foods In Season

No matter where you live in the world, foods can be found in season. Certain meats and obviously fresh fruits and vegetables from your local farmers are not only great for you, but when in season, much cheaper! This is a simple way to save a few bucks, and at the same time hold fast to the Z Diet's recommendation of all the fruits and vegetables you want! While we are on the topic of saving money, when you are able, buy in bulk and stick to store brand canned and packaged goods. These are a lot nicer to the wallet than a lot of the name brand identicals.

Your Condition when you go to Food Shop

I am not going to tell you how to dress or do your hair here. I am going to make a few suggestions for your belly, however. Make sure it is well fed. Never go to the store hungry. When you shop with your friend Mr. or Ms. Appetite, you tend to purchase a lot of things you not only did not need, but that are caloric dense, sugar and fat filled. These incidentals cost you money – I have read savings up to $30 a shopping trip with the simple act of going to the store with a full belly.

You also want to be sure to plan your meals ahead of time, and buy only what you need while there. This too is a cost saver, and will allow you to stick with your Z Diet long term weight loss plan.

Reading Labels

Reading labels is vital in the Z Diet lifestyle plan. It can be quite confusing, so I am going to spend a few moments explaining it to you.

All labels are required to show the following:

- Serving Size
- Servings per Container
- Calories per Serving
- Nutrient Amounts per Serving and % daily values:
    - Fat, saturated fat, trans fat, cholesterol
    - Sodium, carbs, protein, sugars, fiber
- The following nutrients as % daily values:
    - Vitamin A
    - Vitamin C
    - Calcium
    - Iron
- List of ingredients by weight

To get a good grasp of what you are about to purchase or swallow, you need to look at each and every one of these items to ensure you know your food! I will provide you with a simple systematic way to glance at a label and know whether you should put it in your shopping cart, or toss it back on the shelf.

First: start at the top and work down. I look at the serving size so I can relate how much actual food is being 'labeled' below. In this case, the serving size is two crackers. The next line tells me how many Servings per Container are in the box or can. This will be important if you take it home and polish off the whole thing during one episode of your favorite TV show. Next, look at Calories per Serving. This tells us that two crackers (the serving size) have 60 calories. So if I eat 4 crackers, I just quickly consumed 120 calories, and so on. Remember how much exercise it takes to burn 120 calories off? Here is where I make my first judgment on this food item. If I look at the calories and realize that, in just a few servings of this item I have to get back to caloric neutral with a lot of exercise, likely a lot more than I have time for, I put it back on the shelf. A simple rule of thumb: If one serving has 60 or more calories, I toss it. If it has fewer, let's move down the label:

Nutrient Amounts per Serving and % daily values are next. The % daily values I would ignore, because unless you are on exactly a 2000 calorie a day diet, who cares. It gets too confusing. I give this

Nutrition Facts
Serving Size 2 crackers (14 g)
Servings Per Container About 21

Amount Per Serving
Calories 60 Calories from Fat 15

	% Daily Value*
Total Fat 1.5g	2%
Saturated Fat 0g	0%
Trans Fat 0g	
Cholesterol 0mg	0%
Sodium 70mg	3%
Total Carbohydrate 10g	3%
Dietary Fiber Less than 1g	3%
Sugars 0g	
Protein 2g	

Vitamin A 0% • Vitamin C 0%
Calcium 0% • Iron 2%

* Percent Daily Values are based on a 2,000 calorie diet. Your daily values may be higher or lower depending on your calorie needs:

	Calories:	2,000	2,500
Total Fat	Less than	65g	80g
Sat Fat	Less than	20g	25g
Cholesterol	Less than	300mg	300mg
Sodium	Less than	2400mg	2400mg
Total Carbohydrate		300g	375g
Dietary Fiber		25g	30g

whole section a glance and make some judgments.

1. How much fat does it have per serving? I know the total calories per serving are fewer than 60 by now or I would have thrown it out,

but where are those calories coming from? If the fat value is high, greater than 5 g per serving, it gets tossed, as that is very caloric dense, and likely not going to be that satisfying for my need to chew. If there are a lot of trans fats, it gets tossed as well, as those are certainly not part of my long term plan. Cholesterol – who cares – ignore it.

2. What is the sodium content? If this is greater than 200 mg per serving, I toss it as well. We do not need a lot of salt confounding our life long quest for health and weight control.

3. How much sugar is there? So far, if the total calories are acceptable and fat is less than 5 grams per serving, sodium is less than 200 mg per serving, what is the sugar content? If the sugar content exceeds 7 grams per serving, move on to the next item. It too is likely caloric dense and better to avoid.

4. What is the protein content? I am probably not going to get a lot of quality protein in something I find in a box, but a few of the canned goods and dairy, for example, are excellent sources of protein, and therefore, by the time the food label meets all of my other requirements listed above, the amount of protein will likely be acceptable, no matter what the number of grams per serving is.

Finally we get toward the bottom. Skip the nutrients as % daily values including Vitamin A, Vitamin C, Calcium, and Iron. You are not likely going to get a substantial amount of any of these nutrients from something with a label on it.

I would look at the List of ingredients by weight, as more of an interest. They list the heaviest items down to the lighter items in order. So if your first item listed is High Fructose Corn Syrup, you can rest assured that what you are holding is nothing more than High Fructose Corn Syrup with a few other thing there for color and/or texture. I might consider tossing this one as well...

Other label stuff of 'weight'

Labels can also be tricky if you were not to take the time to read them as I described above. Let me give you some examples: When a food source claims something to do with calories, fat, or any other thing of importance (especially while following the Z Diet), it must meet the

FDA and RDA's standards for truth in labeling. So if they claim something is Low Calorie, it must have fewer than 40 calories per serving.

I have listed them out in an easy to read format in terms of a primary reference point (the first one being **Calories**) and then given the meaning of each indication, or more likely advertisement, listed on your food source as a way to get you to buy it.

- **Calories**
    - **Low calorie** means fewer than 40 calories per serving
    - **Reduced calorie** means 25% lower in calories *than regular product.* Be careful with this one. If the original product was a 500 calorie phenomenon, you're saving a whopping 125 calories, but still getting 375!
    - **Calorie free** means fewer than 5 calories per serving. You could still manage 75 servings and get yourself in trouble…
- **Fat**
    - **Low fat** means less than 3 grams of fat per serving
    - **Fat free** means less than .5 grams of fat per serving

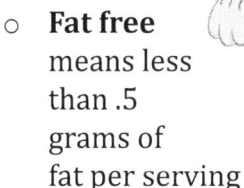

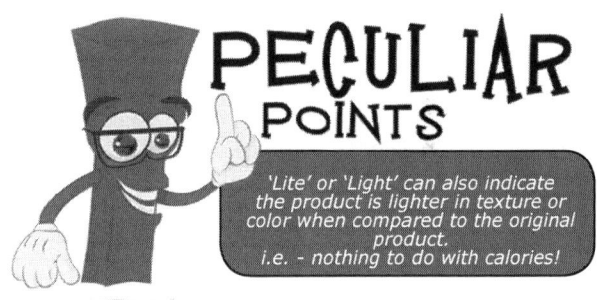

    PECULIAR POINTS
    *'Lite' or 'Light' can also indicate the product is lighter in texture or color when compared to the original product.
    i.e. - nothing to do with calories!*

    - **Low Saturated Fat** means less than 1 gram of saturated fat per serving AND less than .5grams of trans fat per serving
- **Meat and Poultry**
    - **Lean meat and poultry** means less than 10 g fat per

serving, and less than 4.5 grams saturated and trans fat per serving, and less than 95 mg cholesterol per serving

- **Extra Lean meat and poultry** means less than 5 g fat per serving, and less than 2 grams saturated and trans fat per serving, and less than 95 mg cholesterol per serving

- **Sugar**

    - **Sugar Free** means less than .5 grams of sugar per serving

Occasionally labels will make claims like being "Light" or "Healthy" – this is what them mean:

- **Light**

    - Means it must have 1/3 fewer calories than the original product. The same rule mentioned above applies: how many calories does the original product have?

    - Light can mean it has one-half the fat of the original, which is good…

    - Light can also mean the product, when compared to the original simply is **lighter in texture or color** indicating *nothing* about the calories…

    - Light can also simply indicate that, compared to the original product, the amount of Sodium (Na+) is decreased by 50%

- **Healthy**

    - Simply means it is low in fat (trans, saturated, cholesterol) and low in sodium with at least 10% daily values for vitamins A, C, Iron, Calcium, protein, and fiber

- **Good source of**

    - Provides at least 10% of the daily value of a particular vitamin or nutrient per serving

- **High in**
    - Provides at least 20% of the daily value of a specified nutrient/serving

You might notice a few other acronyms listed on your food label. I have listed them below, so you would know what each of them means if/when you run into them:

Dietary Reference Intakes

- **Recommended Dietary Allowances (RDA)**
    - The daily nutrient intake level that meets the needs of 97% of healthy people in a particular stage of life and gender group.
- **Adequate Intake (AI)**
    - The daily nutrient intake level assumed to be adequate when scientific data is lacking to recommend a RDA
- **Estimated Average Requirements (EAR)**
    - The daily nutrient intake estimated to meet the requirements of half of the healthy people in a particular life stage and gender group. EAR values form the scientific basis for which the RDA's are set.
- **Tolerable Upper Intake levels (UL)**
    - The highest daily nutrient intake level that likely poses no risk of toxicity to nearly all healthy people in a particular life stage and gender group.
- **Acceptable Daily Intake (ADI)**
    - Estimated amount of sweetener consumed daily over a lifetime w/o any adverse events

Acupuncture and Hypnotherapy, two alternatives for weight reduction, have some excellent data supporting their use in weight loss and long term weight loss maintenance!

FAT FACTS

As you can tell, reading labels can be a bit tricky, but it is certainly worth your time to do so and part of the Z Diet lifestyle plan! In our next section, I am going to discuss medication and approaching your health care provider about fine tuning of some of your medications and/or the removal or addition of some to help with your long term weight loss maintenance program.

11

Medications And Weightloss

Until very recently, I was the last weight loss doctor to prescribe medication, a true hard-liner if you will. But my view has changed dramatically, and I am becoming more and more aware of the benefits of some of the drugs available out there, especially for long term weight loss. I am also very aware of all of the medications that inhibit people's ability to lose weight, even when weight loss would be much better for them (and, in a lot of cases, cure them of the reason they need the drug in the first place).

Medications are a part of life, like it or not. As the Z Diet is a lifestyle, I have to consider the fact that medication is a part of a lot of people's lives. It is most certainly needed in a variety of situations, and though the argument could be raised that proper eating and daily exercise could have, should have, and would have prevented a lot of the reasons people take medications, that is neither here or there. Fighting weight gain after loss and obesity in and of itself is a chronic life long process. It is even considered a chronic disease in a number of medical minds. Medications are utilized for every other chronic disease, why not prevention of weight gain?

As with everything in life, to appease the lawyers, I must add another disclaimer right now.

Medications and all drugs for that matter can be dangerous without proper consultation with your doctor. This chapter is not intended to replace medical advice. Nothing can compare to a face-to-face conversation with your doctor in relation to your health. If you are sick, or suspect you are sick, you need to see your doctor. If you are taking prescription medication, talk to your health care provider before making any changes to your medication regimen. Talk to your doctor if you have an interest in learning more about how medication may be affecting you and your ability to lose weight. Never purchase prescription drugs from the Internet, and be sure to discuss dietary and exercise changes with your doctor before implementing.

I am going to approach this chapter in three sections. The first will be a little history of medications used for weight loss and the uphill battle that many face with the weight loss drugs. The second will be on some of the more popular weight loss drugs and their indications for both short term and long term weight loss, and finally, I will cover some drugs that inhibit weight loss, and some whose use can even put the weight back on. I will not be covering a number of drugs that may be construed as 'on the edge' or 'underground'.

History Of Weight Loss Drugs

Without question, the mad and frantic search for "the weight loss pill" has been in full swing since the first pharmaceutical company opened its doors. As this is obvious, I am not going to cover it. The history I want to cover concerns the dispute over the weight loss drugs both in the public and professional domain.

It is most unfortunate, but the majority of the public feels that "obesity is a disorder of willpower", and therefore the weight loss drugs do nothing for you in the long run. And with this, they equate badness. In the professional world the majority of medical opinion focuses on the fact that the drugs must not work, because weight eventually plateaus on the drug and once a person stops using the drug, the weight comes back. The logic behind this is belief of a true therapeutic failure and reflects failure of the drug. I have been guilty of this very stance, one I have since recanted. It is a most unfortunate error in logic as I, and I am sure every primary care doctor out there, see people with hypertension (high blood pressure) whose blood pressure plateaus, and we think nothing of increasing the dose or adding another medication. Try doing that with weight loss drugs...the medical boards will likely be knocking on some doors and sending nasty-o-grams.

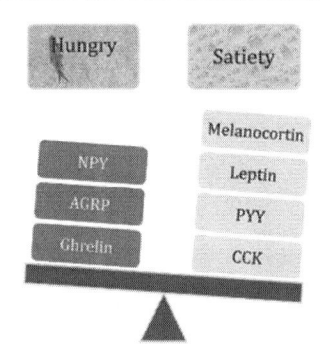

The answer is obvious to me now. Use the drugs as *part* of the solution. Don't rely on them to be *the* solution. The majority of doctors who write prescriptions for dietary drugs do simply that: they write prescriptions for the drugs, with no mention of diet or exercise or the infamous "what's next?" question. Hence part of the bad rap the drugs get. The drugs also find themselves "guilty by association" as the majority of the popular appetite suppressants are what we call sympathomimetic amines, closely related to Amphetamine (speed, crank, meth, etc.).

So we have both public and professional opinion that together give a very negative radiance to the weight loss drugs. But the medical professionals in the area of weight loss, The American Society of Bariatric Physicians (ASBP), say that weight loss drugs are part of the solution. Their approach to weight loss is four fold: correct any underlying metabolic problem, individualize food and exercise plans, provide micronutrient support, and use the anti-obesity medications as indicated.

Even though some negative light has been shown on the obesity drugs, a number of governing medical bodies have recommendations for use of the drugs based on a BMI greater than 30 or a BMI greater than 27 with co-morbidities (such as blood pressure, diabetes, sleep apnea, etc.) These include, but are not limited to: American Association of Clinical Endocrinologist, National Institutes of Health, American Medical Association, and the American Gastroenterology Association.

The recommendations for use of the drugs are much broader with the ASBP and they include: BMI of 30, BMI of 27 with 1 co-morbidity, current body weight of 120% after documented "normal" weight after age 18, body fat percentage of 30% in females and 25% in males, an elevated waist to hip ratio and the presence of at least one co-morbid conditions caused by excessive weight.

The drugs themselves have a variety of goals, and, though beyond the scope of this book to cover each drug and its mechanism of action (other than the common ones I will describe in a minute here) they all work primarily work on one or more of the following:

- Increase Satiety
- Decrease Hunger
- Inhibit gastric emptying
- Decrease Food Intake
- Stimulate Thermogenesis
- Inhibit Lipids
- Decrease Food Absorption

A number of drugs have been studied in all of these areas, a lot of them relying on modification or mimicking the gut and brain hormones that control all of the above. To date, there are only six drugs FDA approved for weight loss, four of the six being appetite suppressants.

A few of the Weight loss Drugs

I will briefly cover a few of the more common drugs used for weight loss, both the FDA approved ones and the ones we use off label (i.e. we use them for weight loss but the FDA has not given an indication for weight loss). Of interesting side note; to meet the FDA's requirement to be considered a weight loss drug, the drug itself, with all other variables removed needs to cause a 5% weight reduction. So if you weigh 300 pounds, and you take a drug and lose 15 pounds, that drug could qualify for FDA weight loss indication. That is not very much, obviously, but may be of some benefit for long term weight loss maintenance.

Agents to decrease hunger

All of these agents are sympathomimetic amines, closely related to Amphetamine, as mentioned above. All of the drugs are similar in their side effects such as a rapid heart rate, anxiety, nervousness, etc. and all of them are contraindicated in people with a history of drug abuse, while using anti-depressants, history of eating disorders or seizure disorder, glaucoma, extremes of age and of course, pregnancy and lactation.

There are four that are FDA approved; Phentermine, Diethylpropion, Phendimetrazine, Benzphetamine. As they are very similar, I will only cover the most popular one, Phentermine. Phentermine also goes by the names: Adipex-P, Ionamin, Obenix, Obephen, Oby-Cap, Oby-Trim, Panshape M, Phentercot, Phentride, Pro-Fast HS, Pro-Fast SA, Pro-Fast SR, Teramine, and Zantryl, and likely others, but I got sick of trying to spell these correctly!

It had a bad rap for a few years due to its combination drug buddy Fenfluramine in Phen – Fen®. Fenfluramines metabolite, norfenfluramine, is the actual culprit in this combination, not the Phentermine. Some of the other concerns with the medication are that it may be addictive. Most would agree that addiction rides the coat tail of Dopamine in the brain (the feel *really* good chemical). Phentermine does not have a methyl group on the side chain with the nitrogen group and therefore has very little, if any, affinity for dopamine receptors. One of the other primary concerns is that it could potentially raise blood pressure. In my experience, there may be a transient rise in blood pressure, especially if someone were to start at the full dose (which you should not – it should be tapered up slowly). From a pharmacologic standpoint, Phentermine does not bind to alpha receptors, and therefore should not affect blood pressure. I have a feeling that the occasional short term rise in blood pressure experienced by some may be due to norepinephrine release (another sympathomimetic amine) when people first start taking the drug, but this is transient.

Phentermine is a great drug for appetite control. The following statement might not be very popular, but it is good for both short term and long term usage. The FDA has stated, as has the Physicians' Desk Reference (a politically controlled periodical if there ever was one) that

Phentermine should only be used, at a maximum, for three months or 90 days. That would make it a weight loss drug, not a weight maintenance drug – correct? I feel it should be and can be used for both. Here is how I would suggest it be used for long term weight loss maintenance: use the drug as needed, on bad days, or when bad temptations rear their ugly head. You are doing wonderfully on the Z Diet, but you have a Christmas party coming up, and are scared to death because you know your co-worker, Mrs. Jones, makes the most delicious, downright malevolent sugar cookies and you will not be able to help yourself when they call your name – follow the suggestions in Appendix III and pop one-half of a Phentermine tablet.

Without question, Phentermine is not for everyone. You need to talk to your doctor or a doctor of Bariatric Medicine to decide if it can be part of your Z Diet long term weight loss maintenance plan.

The next agent to discuss in this section also could be considered one that stimulates thermogenesis, or actually burns fat. It is called Sibutramine or Meridia® , and it is a Selective Norepinephrine Receptor Inhibitor or SNRI. SNRI also inhibits dopamine reuptake, so the potential for addiction is there. The FDA has approved its usage for one year, and it may be of benefit for long term weight loss maintenance. It is contraindicated for a variety of reasons including being on MAO inhibitors, Phentermine, anti-depressant drugs (SSRI's), and a number of pain medications including methadone, meperidine, fentanyl, and others.

I occasionally use this drug, but unfortunately, so many patients have contraindications to its use, my experience is limited. Once again: talk to your doctor to see if this drug may be of benefit to you for long term weight loss maintenance.

Agents to decrease fat absorption

Orlistat ®, also called Xenical® by prescription and Alli® over the counter is a gastric and pancreatic lipase inhibitor that prevents absorption of 1/3 of ingested fat in your diet. Studies show minimal weight loss with these agents – anywhere between 6 to 9 pounds vs. 4 pounds on placebo in most studies. That is not much – especially when you look at the trade off: incontinence of stools and oily spotting in your shorts!

Orlistat is the only weight loss medication approved for kids 12 years of age and older. Some of the side effects mentioned above are partially attenuated with the use of fibers in the diet such as glucomannan, inulin, or psyllium husk.

I personally like my patients. To prescribe something for them that gives them incontinence of stools and oily spotting in their underwear is not something I would do to people I like! That is all I have to say about this drug...

Off Label use of Drugs for Long Term Weight Loss Maintenance

There are a large number of drugs used off label for weight loss, but can any of them be used for weight loss maintenance? In considering the drugs I would cover here, I kept in mind a few primary things:

- Cost – how much does the drug cost, and will you have to mortgage your house to stay on it? If so, it is not listed here.
- Side effects – are the potential risks worth the benefits in long term weight loss maintenance? This one took some consideration, as having a lot of fat on your body far outweighs a lot of the drug risks for your longevity and what you have to deal with day-to-day!
- Convenience – If you have to take the drug five times a day to get anything from it in your lifestyle plan, it's not realistic! I only included it if it would work in the most hectic of schedules!

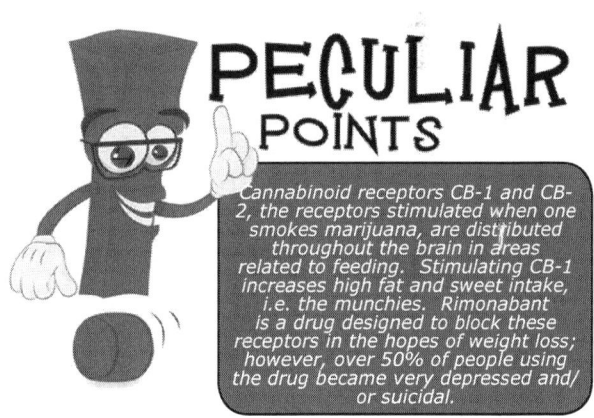

PECULIAR POINTS

Cannabinoid receptors CB-1 and CB-2, the receptors stimulated when one smokes marijuana, are distributed throughout the brain in areas related to feeding. Stimulating CB-1 increases high fat and sweet intake, i.e. the munchies. Rimonabant is a drug designed to block these receptors in the hopes of weight loss; however, over 50% of people using the drug became very depressed and/or suicidal.

Bupropion (Wellbutrin SR, Zyban, Wellbutrin XL)

Bupropion is a norepinephrine and dopamine reuptake inhibitor (NDRI). It was found indirectly, that, while being treated for depression, people lost weight on the drug. It works about the same as

Sibutramine, but costs much less and does not have any dopamine properties (therefore non-addictive). Side effects are similar, and it is a great agent to use in substitution of some of the other anti-depressants (see below). Two good multicenter trials (Jain et al. 2002 and Anderson et al. 2002) showed good effects at 300 and 400 mg of the SR version a day at 24 weeks showing a 7.2% and 10.1% of total body weight loss respectively. As far as long term weight loss maintenance, I think it is an excellent adjunct to the Z Diet. Request the SR version, as in my experience, taking it twice a day really helps the appetite control vs. the XL versions which is once a day (and the SR version is cheaper!).

Bupropion is not for everyone. You need to talk to your doctor or a doctor of Bariatric Medicine to decide if it can be part of your Z Diet long term weight loss maintenance plan.

Metformin (Glucophage)

Metformin is a very commonly used drug for insulin resistance and diabetes. It works by reducing hepatic glucose production, increasing insulin sensitivity, and decreasing absorption from the GI tract. Its primary side effects that I see are some belly disturbance that seems to abate with time. You always have to let it be known you are on the drug because of some serious adverse reactions with IV contrast, for example, if you needed a CT scan.

A number of doctors use this drug as an adjunct for weight loss; however, it really does not help with weight loss *directly*. In the Diabetes Prevention Study, the Metformin group lost 2.5% of body weight over the 3.2 years of follow up. Recall, to be considered a weight loss drug it needs to help you lose 5% of your weight. To use real numbers, if you weighed 200 pounds, your net weight loss thanks to Metformin would be 5 pounds. However, notice I said *direct* weight loss above!

If you are following the Z Diet, especially if you are metabolically challenged, Metformin is a wonderful addition to your long term plan. With its effects on insulin sensitivity, if you are eating and exercising daily as discussed in the Z Diet, your weight loss will be aided with Metformin.

As with all the medications, Metformin is not for everyone. You need to talk to your doctor or a doctor of Bariatric Medicine to decide if it can be part of your Z Diet long term weight loss maintenance plan.

Spironolactone

Spironolactone is a diuretic used for a number of things including edema associated with excessive aldosterone excretion; hypertension; primary hyperaldosteronism; hypokalemia; cirrhosis of liver accompanied by edema or ascites. We use it off label for Poly Cystic Ovarian Syndrome (PCOS) - an insulin related condition, as it helps with excessive hair (hirsutism) and even helps a little with female acne.

Spironolactone does *nothing* for weight loss! It does nothing to your fat cells, your energy expenditure, or any other facet of weight loss. It is a diuretic, so you will hear and likely read on the internet about it causing weight loss, but it is all water weight, as discussed in the diuresis section of Quick Weight Loss Solutions.

I am mentioning it here, because it has some uses once again in PCOS, and the majority of gals with PCOS have some extra weight/fat, but it is also useful during the luteal phase of the menstrual cycle. As we discussed in an earlier chapter, this is the time of month when energy expenditure increases, as does your eating, particularly the high fat and high sugar stuff. Adding magnesium is your first step, followed in short order by utilizing Spironolactone in low doses, the week or two before menstruation.

I cannot tell you exactly how it benefits the food cravings, but it does seem to work, and a lot of Bariatric doctors use it in just this manner.

As the record is obviously broken: talk to your doctor or a doctor of Bariatric Medicine to decide if it can be part of your Z Diet long term weight loss maintenance plan.

Bupropion and Naltrexone

Bupropion you will recognize from above. Naltrexone is a pure opioid receptor antagonist. In other words it blocks the effects of opioids such as morphine and heroin. We use it in medicine to treat overdoses as well as help people with alcoholism and drug addiction. It has recently gotten a lot of press for a number of other conditions, but that is beyond our discussion here. Both bupropion and naltrexone have been shown individually to induce weight loss. Bupropion seems to work better on its own for weight loss, but Naltrexone (particularly the SR version) potentiates the effects of bupropion; thus, this synergistic combination has the potential for good long term weight loss control.

The naltrexone-bupropion combination is designed to promote hypothalamic proopiomelanocortin (a brain hormone that causes satiety) activity, which reduces appetite and stimulates energy expenditure. A few early studies show some good results, but as it falls in this section of the book, the FDA has yet to approve its use for weight loss.

There are obvious concerns with any drug therapy, including side effects, interactions, contraindications, etc., and you should talk to your doctor if you are interested in learning more.

Vitamin D

Vitamin D has also received a lot of press lately. It has made its way into the Holy Grail of medicine, as a study a week comes out exploiting another benefit of high levels in the body, and the horrors of low levels. There have been a number of studies on low levels being associated with a fat problem, but the chicken and the egg question once again rears its head i.e. does a low vitamin D levels attribute to obesity, or does obesity cause low vitamin D levels. It is true however that there are vitamin D receptors on fat cells and a deficiency of vitamin D seems to allow the fat cell to grow.

I can tell you that when levels are low, replacing them with a loading dose over a few weeks then maintaining them with an adequate daily dose does assist with the big picture. I cannot attribute direct long term weight loss maintenance with Vitamin D, but it seems to be part of it.

The reason it is in the medication chapter, as I am sure you are aware you can purchase it over the counter, is because getting your levels checked requires a doctor's visit and doing a proper loading dose with either high dose oral medications or injections is also best done under the direction of a physician.

Testosterone

I briefly mentioned Testosterone under the Hormonally Challenged section of the book as it related to Andropause in men. Now let me share some information in regard to proper levels and weight loss maintenance.

Testosterone can be of benefit for long term weight loss maintenance in both men and women for a variety of reasons: first, as you recall from the chapter on Understanding Dieting, testosterone levels are one of the first things to go with caloric restriction. As with any long term weight loss lifestyle, you need to exercise daily. Testosterone will help with your recovery so you can get up and do it again tomorrow. It also keeps you in an anabolic state (out of catabolism) to protect your muscles for both their look and function. It provides a mental boost and a healthy aggression to keep you focused, increases energy and strength, builds bone mass improves sexual function and libido, and in proper doses improves your cholesterol profile. All of these things and more assist in your goals of long term weight loss maintenance. Testosterone also has an added benefit in the metabolically challenged, as it has been show to help control if not be directly involved in insulin resistance reversal. I have seen in clinical practice notable improvements in diabetes blood sugar with the initiation of testosterone therapy as well.

Testosterone in and of itself does not cause fat loss. Even in extremely well shaped athletes using anabolic steroids such as Testosterone, their fat loss and leanness are due to their diet and exercise program. I mention it here because I am continually amazed at how many people have low levels and have the subjective complaints to accompany said levels. Testosterone replacement in these men and women can be of great benefit for long term weight loss maintenance.

Testosterone is a controlled prescription drug and needs to be tested, administered, and followed up by a doctor competent in hormone replacement.

Progesterone

As you recall from our discussion of the hormonally challenged, following ovulation, women enter the luteal phase of their cycle, where estrogen starts to decrease and progesterone starts to rise. This causes an increase in energy expenditure and they burn more calories in the luteal phase of their cycle. I also mentioned it is difficult to decipher if this increase in energy expenditure is a result of estrogen going down, or progesterone elevating. I have a feeling it is both, but I will occasionally use progesterone in the luteal phase of a woman's cycle, as it seems to help with the long term weight loss maintenance during this time of increased hunger.

Similar to Spironolactone, I have women use it from day 15 of their cycle to day 25 (assuming they are on a regular 28 day cycle). Dose, side effects, etc. all need to be discussed individually. Progesterone is definitely a consideration for long term weight loss control.

Drugs that are best avoided in long term weight loss

A number of very commonly prescribed drugs can actually inhibit weight loss and are guilty of causing weight gain. I am going to cover a few of the more common ones here, as well as provide some potential alternatives. To re-iterate: do not change your medications on your own! If you happen to be on one of them I mention, talk to your doctor about a workable alternative for you.

When I look at a drug, I consider all aspects of the drug, as all doctors do, but due to my profession, I also consider whether the drug I am looking at is weight positive, weight neutral, or weight negative. Weight positive drugs can cause weight gain, weight neutral drugs do not cause weight gain or loss, and weight negative drugs actually cause weight loss.

In considering the best way to approach this, I decided to list a few of the medical problems readers might have, then list a few of the common drugs utilized to treat those disorders under the sub-heading of weight positive or weight negative in a chart like format. Obviously, these are not all inclusive lists. At the most, I would hope they would give you the opportunity to discuss with your doctor any medication's side effects, in particular with regard to its effects on your long term weight loss plan.

Hypertension (elevated blood pressure)

Weight Positive Drugs	Weight Neutral or Negative Drugs/Alternatives
Beta Blockers: Atenolol (Tenormin) Metoprolol (Lopressor, Toprol XL) Levobunolol (Betagan) Nadolol (Corgard) Propranolol (Ineral, Innopran XL) **Thiazide Diuretics:** Chlorothiazide (Diuril) Hydrochlorothizazide (HCTZ) Metolazone (Zaroxolyn) **Loop Diuretics:** Bumetanide (Bumex) Ethacrynic acid (Edecrin) Furosemide (Lasix) Torsemide (Demadex) **Calcium Channel Blockers:** Amlodipine (Norvasc) Diltiazem (Cardizem LA, Dilacor XR) Felodipine (Plendil) Isradipine (DynaCirc CR) Nicardipine (Cardene, Cardene SR) Nifedipine (Procardia, Procardia XL, Adalat CC) Nisoldipine (Sular) Verapamil (Calan Verelan, Covera-HS) **Alpha-Adrenergic Blockers:** Doxazosin (Cardura) Prazosin (Minipress) Terazosin (Hytrin) Tamsulosin (Flomax) Alfuzosin (Uroxatral) Of note – A few Beta Blockers do not have the weight positive effect, including those with alpha activity.	**ACE Inhibitors:** Benazepril hydrochloride (Lotensin) Captopril (Capoten) Enalapril maleate (Vasotec) Fosinopril sodium (Monopril) Lisinopril (Prinivil, Zestril) Moexipril (Univasc) Quinapril hydrochloride (Accupril) Ramipril (Altace) Trandolapril (Mavik) **Angiotensin II receptor blockers** Losartan potassium (Cozaar) Valsartan (Diovan) Irbesartan (Avapro)

Diabetes

Weight Positive Drugs	Weight Neutral or Negative Drugs/ Alternatives
Thiazolidinediones: Rosiglitazone (Avandia) Pioglitazone (Actos) **Sulfonylureas:** Glimepriide (Amaryl) Glipizide (Glucotrol, Glucotrol XL) Glybuide (DiaBeta, Micronase)	**Biguanide:** Metformin (Glucophage) **Incretin Mimetics:** Exenatide (Byetta)

Depression

Weight Positive Drugs	Weight Neutral or Negative Drugs/ Alternatives
Tricyclic Anti-depressants: Amitriptyline Amoxapine Desipramine (Norpramin) Doxepin (Sinequan) Imipramine (Tofranil, Tofranil-PM) Nortriptyline (Pamelor) Protriptyline (Vivactil) Trimipramine (Surmontil) **SSRI's** Fluoxetine (Prozac, Prozac Weekly) Paroxetine (Paxil, Paxil CR, Pexeva) Sertraline (Zoloft) **MAOI's:** Selegiline (Emsam) Isocarboxazid (Marplan)	**NDRI's:** Bupropion (WellButrin) **SNRI's:** Venlafaxine (Effexor, Effexor XR) Duloxetine (Cymbalta)

PECULIAR POINTS

The Ten Commandments contain 297 words.
The Bill of Rights is 463 words.
Lincoln's Gettysburg Address contains 266 words.
A recent federal directive to regulate the price of cabbage contains 26,911 words.
This book is just over 55,000 words.
Therefore, it can be concluded that the most important documents in the world are short and to the point, and the long winded documents are written by the government and weight loss professionals!

Chronic Headaches (prophylaxis)

Weight Positive Drugs	Weight Neutral or Negative Drugs/ Alternatives
Beta Blockers: Metoprolol (Lopressor, Toprol XL) Propranolol (Ineral, Innopran XL) **MAOI's:** Selegiline (Emsam) Isocarboxazid (Marplan)	**Anticonvulsants:** Toperimate (Topamax)

Sleep Disorders

Weight Positive Drugs	Weight Neutral or Negative Drugs/ Alternatives
Tricyclic Anti-depressants: Amitriptyline Amoxapine Desipramine (Norpramin) Doxepin (Sinequan) Imipramine (Tofranil, Tofranil-PM) Nortriptyline (Pamelor) Protriptyline (Vivactil) Trimipramine (Surmontil)	**Nonbenzodiazepine Hypnotic:** Zolpidem (Ambien) Eszopiclone (Lunesta)

Chronic Pain (i.e. fibromyalgia)

Weight Positive Drugs	Weight Neutral or Negative Drugs/ Alternatives
Tricyclic Anti-depressants: Amitriptyline Amoxapine Desipramine (Norpramin) Doxepin (Sinequan) Imipramine (Tofranil, Tofranil-PM) Nortriptyline (Pamelor) Protriptyline (Vivactil) Trimipramine (Surmontil)	**SNRI's:** Venlafaxine (Effexor, Effexor XR) Duloxetine (Cymbalta)

Allergies of all kinds (seasonal, itchy skin, etc)

Weight Positive Drugs	Weight Neutral or Negative Drugs/ Alternatives
Antihistamines Clemastine Diphenhydramine (Benadryl) Doxylamine (most commonly used as an OTC sedative) Loratadine Desloratadine Fexofenadine Pheniramine Cetirizine Ebastine Promethazine Chlorpheniramine Levocetirizine Quetiapine (antipsychotic) Meclizine (most commonly used as an antiemetic) Dimenhydrinate (most commonly used as an antiemetic)	**Avoid allergens! Stay well hydrated and eat right and exercise daily!**

Another potential weight positive drug class is the drugs made for reflux disease or Gastrointestinal Reflux Disease (GERD). Both the Proton Pump Inhibitors (PPI's) and the Histamine 2 (H2) blockers may contribute to weight gain. The mechanisms are many, but needless to say part of the reasons for the need of these medicines is late night eating and crappy diets! Cut those two out, lose weight, (see previous...) and you will likely not need them!

In summary, this was a very simple review of a few medications and their potential role in long term weight loss maintenance. If you have any questions about anything in this chapter, or the Z Diet in general, I encourage you to discuss them with your primary care provider.

12

Summary

Hopefully, by now you have a good grasp of what the Z Diet and its connotations in long term weight loss look like. Before I simply review each step for you with a paragraph or two, let me add one quick blurb on why I am well know for saying "there is no such things as a bad food, just bad eating plans/diets".

I most certainly in favor of good, quality, low processed, high fiber, water, and air filled foods, with emphasis on lean meats and dairy, nuts and seeds, and all of the great stuff the good Lord has given us to eat. There is a reason I do not jump start people on to the good foods, and let them continue on with the foods they are use to as they start an eating plan (or maintain one). When you have written as many diets and eating plans as I have and worked with thousands of people in the area of weight loss, you begin to realize the absolute amount of change that must take place in their lives so they can reach their goals. You think quitting tobacco is hard? In one fell swoop, try changing your diet, fitting exercise into your daily schedule, relearning how to shop, breaking habits like eating before bed with the TV on, etc. One way I have found that is very beneficial to people is to start this process by teaching them the philosophy of The Z Diet. They start by adding breakfast to their day, eat according to their schedules, cut their carbohydrates out by mid afternoon, make sure they have protein at each meal, etc. They do that with the foods they like and are accustom to. I tell them *how* to eat, not *what* to eat. When people do this, a fascinating thing occurs: they start feeling better. They get more energy. They sleep better. They start to lose fat. They increase their strength. In other words, they start to use foods, to their benefit, that other diet plans would consider horrific. They suffer fewer adverse food reactions (like getting fat), even with less than ideal foods. *They reset their baseline.* Once this baseline has been reset, they start *seeking out better foods!* They decrease their visits to the fast food establishments; they start reading labels and avoiding trans fats and excessive sodium. They add extra fiber to their diet. They get healthier! The trick is to use The Z Diet principles first, then start eliminating the less than optimal stuff, and ensure the addition of the really good stuff!

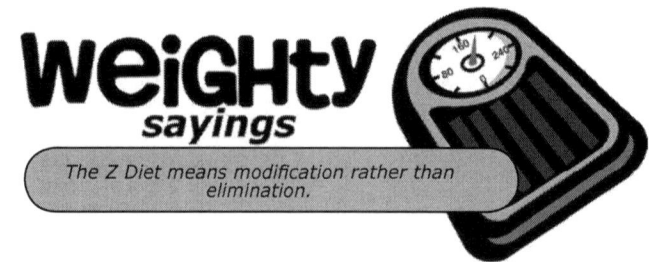

WEIGHTY sayings
The Z Diet means modification rather than elimination.

It really is rather simple and a primary reason I wrote this book. I want to meet people where they are at, and incorporate *lifestyle changes that will last lifelong.* Good eating in general and the Z Diet specifically is a process, not an event! Dieting and quick weight loss is an event, as once you stop; you eventually get your weight back! Real lifelong weight loss maintenance is a process. That process can be summed up with the Z Diet.

So let's review the steps of the Z Diet:

Step One: Lose the weight

Your first step could potentially involve the Z Diet, but more than likely will require strict caloric control with a VLED or a LCD as I discussed in **Quick Weight Loss Approaches** and/or a vigorous exercise program. It is my hope that you adhered to safe practices when you did the more caloric restricted or caloric burning plan, and if you have not undertaken the weight loss, please find a board certified weight loss doctor to help you do so. Now that your weight is off, you can use the Z Diet lifestyle to help keep it off.

Step Two: Know your starting point

Once you have lost the weight, it is important to determine what your *current* starting point is. Are you metabolically challenged, hormonally challenged, after that ultimate body, or do you just want the good health benefits of weight loss maintenance? If you are larger, as defined by percent body fat greater than 35% in females and 25% in males, start living the Z Diet and start to see the benefits (**The Willey Principle**). As you come closer to your goal weight, become more vigilant with calories to ensure you will continue to maintain your new found weight loss. Be sure to track your results, as every time you take a measurement, you have a new starting point. Ideally, follow your body composition to ensure your lean mass is at the very least remaining stable with your long term plan. Based on your answer to this and your current size, you can direct your foods, in particular the macronutrients to your benefit, which brings us to step three:

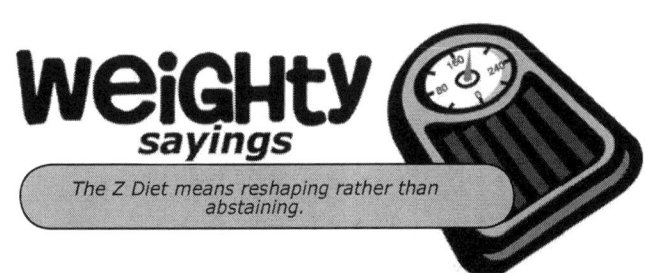

The Z Diet means reshaping rather than abstaining.

Step Three: Understand the macronutrients

Knowing not only what protein, carbohydrate, and fat are but also their caloric density, as well as their importance in your diet for taste, variety, and satiety, is essential in a long term weight loss program. I would encourage you to occasionally re-read the chapter on **The Basics of Foods** as a refresher, as a thorough understanding of them will assist you in your goals.

Step Four: Eat adequate protein

Protein is essential in long term weight loss. A few studies and opinions may vary, but as a weight loss practitioner, I can tell you that this is an important step. Keep adequate protein at every meal using the correct portion sizes as discussed for its benefits in satiety and keeping those muscles filled with fresh amino acids for strength in activities of daily living and everything else life throws at you. Simply take your scale weight in pounds and multiply it times one to get the number of grams of protein you need to be consuming each and every day. Protein has four calories per gram, and most quality protein sources have some fat and carbohydrates in them, so be sure to be aware of your total calories.

Step Five: Become calorie aware

Take a few days and weigh and measure and calculate caloric amounts of your food so you have a rough idea how to size it up in comparison to your hand. Use direct caloric control by avoiding caloric dense foods, and using smaller serving plates and dishes. Eat your larger meals in the following order: water, salad, vegetables, protein, carbohydrates. Avoid dining out if possible and be sure to *know your food!* At all costs and efforts, avoid liquid calories such as fruit juices, pops, energy drinks, sports drinks, etc. These direct caloric control methods are an essential part of the Z Diet!

Step Six: Live the Z lifestyle with indirect caloric control!

I covered a number of things that will assist you in controlling your total caloric intake, indirectly. The mechanisms behind a number of these things reach far beyond simple caloric reduction, but that is topic for another book. Remember to always have your biggest meal in the morning (when you wake up) and the smallest in the evening. Choose the number of meals you eat based on your schedule and what works for you. Use Chrononutrakinetics and Food Timing to optimize your day by keeping your active carbohydrates in your eating plan earlier vs. later. Don't eat before bed so you can wake up hungry and ready for that first meal. Exercise every day with planned exercise activities and remember NEAT and SPA activities – if you have a chance to move, take it!

Be certain to cycle your eating plan based on the factors laid out for you, and never forget the importance of a scheduled or prescription break.

Use some sort of tracking instrument, ideally body composition with your scale weight, but don't forget all the other subjective and objective ways to track your progress.

When you are confined by a schedule, schedule your activity and food as part of that agenda. On days you are not scheduled, be very aware of what you are doing and try to adhere to the lifestyle of the Z Diet, but do not beat yourself up over it.

Step Seven: Follow the shopping guide and learn how to read labels

Simply put; this works and saves you money! Use this shopping guide every time you or a loved one goes to buy food. Learn to read those labels and watch out for subtleties – they can add a lot of calories without your permission!

Step Eight: Work with your doctor to change, adjust, and utilize medication for your long term benefit

Utilize your doctor or a board certified Bariatric physician to help you manage or utilize some medical and pharmacological options for your long term weight loss lifestyle plan. This can be for your initial weight loss and/or your maintenance lifestyle.

Finally:

The Z Diet's application into daily life should be an easy transition for anyone to make. Apply just one of the indirect caloric control options initially, for example, and you will start to notice a difference. Apply them all and I guarantee you will notice a distinction be it in your attempt to lose weight or ideally in your goal to maintain your weight loss. As always, I am excited to meet with anyone reading this book, or at the very least answer some short (please keep them short) emails. One of my greatest joys in life is

MEDICAL MINUTE

If you have ever taken anti-bacterials for an infection, you need to take some pro-biotics. Pro-biotics are the friendly bacteria and are taken for the purpose of re-colonizing areas of the body where they normally would occur. Good bacteria have several functions, including metabolizing foods and certain drugs, absorbing nutrients, and preventing growth of pathogenic (bad) bacteria. One type in particular, Lactobacilli, seems to provide nutritional benefits, including inducing growth factors and increasing the bioavailability of minerals. This can be vital in both weight loss and long term weight loss maintenance.

to see people accomplish something long term, in particular when it comes to their health. With all the talk on the health care problems we have in this country, starting the Z Diet may be one of the answers doctors, insurance companies and individuals are looking for. Health starts with you, and you need to continually work on your health. The Z Diet is a simple way to do just that.

God Bless and the Best in Health and **Z**ellness!

Warren

Appendix I

The Glycemic Index

A lot of attention has been given to the glycemic index – from a stack of books high enough for me to climb on and get to my roof, to full weight loss centers basing their entire philosophy on it. It seems like most things in life (in particular dieting); it has diehard fans who become death-dealers if you disagree with any aspect of it and you have your skeptics who, for whatever reason, think it is bunk. Once again, relying on clinical experience, I seem to find myself in the middle in most circumstances, including the glycemic index. I lean toward the "in favor of" group with the metabolically challenged. And I sway to the other side when it comes to your general healthy person looking for weight loss and your extremely fit individual wanting to better his or her game or physique. Let me give you a little more detail, but first, as always, definitions for clarity.

The glycemic index is a way to rank foods based on how they make your blood sugar rise a few hours after they're eaten. Before its development in the early 1980's, the general thought was a sugar was a sugar, and eating anything that resembled a sugar caused a rapid rise in blood sugar followed in short order by insulin. A few of you likely remember being taught that a complex carbohydrate was/is good, and a simple carbohydrate was/is bad. Research in this area has proven different; that carbohydrates in general have, once eaten, different rates of absorption (based on a number of things I will cover in a second), and, therefore, different responses of blood sugar to their ingestion.

The numbers in the suggested in the glycemic index are percentages with respect to a reference food on a scale where white bread is equal to 100. It is based on a rating system for 50 grams of *available* carbohydrates in the foods consumed. That can be confusing, as a food might weigh 150 grams, but only have 50 grams of *available* carbohydrates, as fiber, for example, is not included. Once the 50 grams of available carbohydrates have been consumed, the blood sugar is recorded and a glycemic index (GI) number is assigned to the food. The GI number is relative to a standard and the number provided is simply a way to classify it. The number really means nothing, other than giving you the ability to compare it to other foods.

The GI is beneficial in helping anyone, in particular the metabolically challenged, to determine foods that raise blood sugar and therefore insulin rapidly, as this has been shown to be detrimental to people with insulin problems. For example: the glycemic index has shown us that simple sugars do not necessarily raise the blood sugar any faster than a few other common foods. A baked potato has a much higher glycemic index than table sugar. Without question, the higher (and more often or longer) blood sugar is elevated, the more concerns with medical and fatness evils. The emblematic vicious cycle.

It is important to understand that the GI value of a food only tells you how quickly blood sugar elevates in response to its consumption. It does not tell you how *much* of that carbohydrate is in a serving of that food. I have had a number of clients stick to the GI like glue in their food choices in hopes of improving their metabolic condition and losing weight. Unfortunately, this meant they did nothing more than avoid foods with high GIs, and eat ad libum all of the lower GI foods without any concern or awareness of calories. There are some benefits to eating nothing but low GI foods, and I will come to that shortly.

Another and likely more important issue concerning the GI is the Glycemic Load (GL). The GL takes into account *quantity* of available carbohydrates. The glycemic load measures the effect of the glycemic index of a food multiplied by its available carbohydrate content in grams, using a standard serving size. Watermelon, a commonly criminalized food for purists of the GI world, has a high GI; however, when looking at the total amounts of carbohydrate available, there are not many there, so watermelon has a low GL.

A simple way to look at it in the big picture is: foods that have a low GL almost always have a low GI. Foods with an intermediate or high GL, range from very low to very high GI.

There are some other variables that affect the GI and GL of foods. These include how much food already resides in your belly at the time you eat. Eating a food after a fast will have a different effect on your blood sugar than eating the same food an hour after having already eaten. How the food was prepared is also critical. Rice, for example, has a much higher GI if you cook it for 20 minutes vs. 5 minutes. Mixing foods together changes the effect on blood sugar, as explained in the insulin section in a previous chapter – **PFFV**! Remember? The amount of processing a food goes through also affects its GI, yet one more reason to avoid the man made stuff.

Your current physical condition also changes the way your blood sugar responds to food. Endurance athletes had a much lower response of their blood sugar than non-trained individuals eating the same foods (breakfast cereal in this study) (1). This is something I see in clinical practice as well (and one of the reasons I ride the fence with recommending the GI to everyone out there). Sounds like chrononutrakinetics does it not? What is the body doing with the foods ingested vs. what is the food doing to the body?

As far as weight loss is concerned, and in particular long term weight loss maintenance, I think the GI and GL can be useful as low GL and GI foods are usually less processed, higher in water, air, and fiber (**PWAF**!). Studies that have looked directly at low GI foods and weight loss always seem to split results. This may be due to the fact that other factors were not accounted for (the amount of protein, for example, as low GI diets tend to be higher in protein and a few studies I have read did not account for the amount of exercise being done). Studies also seem to be conflicting as to whether low GI foods decrease appetite, but I (and I am sure you) have observed that high GI foods increase appetite. Remember that commercial "Bet you cannot eat just one…" so take that one as you will.

One more wrench for your engine: awhile ago I had a thought (dangerous, to say the least, as my wife will acknowledge) concerning the GI. Working with one of my friends as he was preparing for a bodybuilding show, I noticed a few different ways his body was responding to the eating plans I was writing for him. Briefly; due to his schedule he eats frequently with protein at every meal. He has a history of some insulin problems and any quick spikes in insulin are noticeable to him (high self-awareness). I have seen it before, but with other clients with whom my face-to-face contact is limited (they come in for bi-weekly to monthly visits) and he I see every day. We, of course, utilized low glycemic foods, particularly in light of extreme caloric deficits, with intermittent high GI foods such as in post workout meals. Long story short; my observations made me wonder if a particular low GI food, for whatever reason or condition either the body or the food is in, is only a low glycemic food because of a *rapid* insulin response and therefore, sugar never really gets that high? In other words, was the food labeled with a low GI because it was removed from the blood stream so quickly by a high insulin spike? I went on a literature search and I found one article that basically said this is possible (2). This study took two cereals with the same amount of available carbs and showed that the cereal with the low GI had a much more rapid insulin response than the one with the high GI. It was felt that this was due to the protein in the low GI cereal. It is interesting to me, as most athletes know that adding a protein to a carb causes a faster insulin response, and therefore they get more of the benefits of insulin, particularly immediately following exercise (See my book **Better Than Steroids**). So protein lowers the GI of the food, as we have discussed, but is it due to a more rapid response from insulin? What this means consequently for folks with metabolic challenges, or anyone for that matter, I cannot say. I have some thoughts, but as I just told you – that can be dangerous, so I will hold my tongue and my typing fingers for now. As more is learned, I hope to have the opportunity to share!

In summary, the GI and GL can be very useful tools, particularly if you are metabolically challenged. The simple fact to this and the whole concept of the Z Diet and long term weight loss maintenance is it needs to be individualized and tailored to *you*! If you wonder what high GI and GL foods do to your blood sugar, measure it, particularly if you are diabetic. If a low GI diet *does* lower your appetite, then I guess you know the way you need to eat and what foods to focus on. It really comes down to how they affect you.

The following is a simple chart I have published in previous books. It is a simple list of foods and their relative GI. It also includes the optimum time of day when these foods should be eaten. That clarification is nothing more that eating the higher GI foods earlier in the day, and the lower GI foods later – all for optimum blood sugar and insulin control i.e. Food Timing.

1. Mettler S et al. The Influence of the subjects training state on the glycemic index. Eur J of Clin Nutr (2007) Jan;61(1):19-24.

2. Schenk S, Davidson CJ, Zderic TW. Different glycemic indexes of breakfast cereals are not due to glucose entry into blood but to glucose removal by tissue Am J Clin Nutr 2003;78(suppl):742–8.

Simple GI of Common Foods

ANYTIME FOODS:
(Slow inducers of insulin secretion – LOW GI)
Most meats
Most cheeses
Free Carbs

BEFORE 3:00 PM:
(Moderate inducers of insulin secretion- MODERATE GI)
Kidney beans
Black beans
Soymilk
Apricots, dried
Butter beans
Milk, skim
Lima beans, baby, frozen
Fettuccine
Garbanzo beans
Pinto beans
Kellogg's All Bran Fruit 'N Oats
Mars Snicker Bar
Apple juice
Spaghetti, white
Pear, fresh
Navy beans
Tomato soup
Plums
Yogurt, low fat, artificially sweet
Soy-beans (canned)
Peanuts
Soya beans
Rice beans
Green apples
Cherries
Fructose
Peas, dried
Grapefruit
Red lentils
Spaghetti, protein enriched
Milk, full fat

BEFORE NOON:
(Moderate inducers of insulin secretion- MODERATE GI)
All-bran
Peach, fresh
Mars Twix Cookie Bar (Carmel)
Orange
Pears (canned)
Sweet potato
Mars chocolate
Pinto beans (canned)
Macaroni
Linguine
Instant Rice, boiled 1 minute
Sponge Cake
Grapes
Pineapple juice
Peaches (canned)
Instant noodles
Green Peas
Mixed grain bread
Grapefruit juice
Baked beans
High fructose corn syrup
Muffins
Potato, canned
Ice cream
Oatmeal
Hamburger bun
Split pea soup
Pizza, cheese
Pastry
Rice vermicelli
Rice, white
Bran Chex
Honey
Apricots, fresh
Pita bread, white
Power bar
Kellogg's Mini Wheat
Mango

EARLY MORNING:
(Rapid inducers of insulin secretion – HIGH GI)
Rice Krispies
Pretzels
Jellybeans
Post Flakes
Rice cakes
Vanilla Wafers
Coco Pops
Total cereal
Waffles
Donuts
Pumpkins
Cheerios cereal
Puffed Wheat cereal
Potato, boiled, mashed
Rutabaga
Watermelon
Bagel, white
Golden Grahams
Wheat bread, white
Potato, mashed
Cream Of Wheat
Melba toast
Shredded Wheat
Wheat bread, high fiber
Taco shells
Stoned wheat thins
Grape Nuts Cereal
Croissant
Pineapple
Potato, steamed
Sucrose
Macaroni and cheese
Raisins
Apricots, (canned), syrup
Tofu frozen desert, non-dairy
Maltodextrin
Dates
Rice, instant, boiled 6 minutes
Rice Chex
Potatoes, micro waved

Appendix II

Popular Quick Weight Loss Diets

I am attempting to review a few of the most popular diet plans out there in a simple format of positives, negatives, and how they actually work to help you lose weight. I am by no means cutting on them or trying to make my own look good. I have simply summed up some facts that are available in the diet plans. Every one of these has been successful for someone, at the very least for short term weight loss.

The 'how it works' portion is most certainly my opinion, as the diet's success in certain people is attributed to many factors based on the particular diet's system. I am pointing out the reason I think it works, as I reviewed in the introduction.

ABS Diet

Positives:

Lots of good food and promises guys that the girls will clamor all over them.

Negatives:

Very difficult exercise schedule

How it works:

Monotonous eating and tons of exercise (burn the calories).

Ideal Protein Diet

Positives

Rapid short term weight loss. They encourage a lot of protein.

Negatives:

Expensive. Fake food, lots of powders and protein bars and criminalize all sugar. Not realistic long term for your wallet or your weight loss.

How it works:

Lose a lot of water at first, and drink a lot of protein, thereby consuming fewer calories.

Atkins

Positives:

Lots of good meat, dairy and fat!

Negatives:

Not realistic long term.

How it works:

Lose a lot of water at first, and with carbs being criminalized, you eat fewer calories.

French women don't get fat

Positives:

Real food is utilized, including what we think all French people eat: bread, wine, etc.

Negatives:

32% of French women are fat.

How it works:

Decreases your calories by small portion sizes, no snacks, no processed foods.

Deal-A-Meal

Positives:

Utilized like a game to keep you interested. Keeps food simple.

Negatives:

Impossible to use outside the home.

How it works:

Decreases your calories by small portion sizes.

Jenny Craig

Positives:

Great support.

Negatives:

Not real life foods, expensive.

How it works:

Decreases your calories by small portion sizes and gets you to exercise.

The Maple Syrup Diet

Positives:

Fast weight loss, mostly water. Cheap.

Negatives:

Really – who would drink that stuff?

How it works:

Decreases your calories to near nothing and makes you pee a lot.

The Neanderthal Diet (Paleolithic or Stone Age Diet)

Positives:

Lots of meat!

Negatives:

No carbohydrates other than things that can be 'gathered'.

How it works:

Like Atkins, you lose a lot of water at first, and with most carbs being criminalized, you eat fewer calories and start their 5 week exercise plan (i.e. you burn more calories)

Ornish

Positives:

Lots of great vegetables, overall healthy, potential cancer protective.

Negatives:

No meat, oils, nuts. Not realistic long term. Difficult recipes to follow.

How it works:

You eat a lot of caloric light foods (so large amounts, few calories) thereby cutting your calories overall. Encourages daily exercise so you burn more calories.

The Perricone Diet

Positives:

Lots of fish!

Negatives:

Creator is a dermatologist, so of course you have to buy fancy creams and lotions, and supplement bottles that cost more than my car. No proof of weight loss.

How it works:

It doesn't; you get nice skin however!

The Raw Foods Diet

Positives:

Twelve pounds of food a day!

Negatives:

Very time consuming. Encourages sticking things up your back side i.e. colonics.

How it works:

Subtly lowers caloric intake with high bulk foods.

The 3-Hour Diet

Positives:

Good philosophy: No bad food, just bad portions.

Negatives:

No proof that eating every three hours increases metabolism (as discussed in the book).

How it works:

Portion control.

The Zone Diet

Positives:

I like the macronutrient break down, the emphasis on good fatty acids, etc.

Negatives:

Difficult for the mathematically challenged and therefore a high drop-out rate.

How it works:

Higher protein, good fats, and portion control.

The Pritikin Diet

Positives:

Frequent feedings for those who need that. Encourages low fat, low sodium, high fiber.

Negatives:

Less than 10% of your total daily intake from fat is very hard and impossible long term.

How it works:

With the low fat and daily exercise, this is yet another cut in your calories therefore weight loss.

Nutrisystem

Positives:

No calorie counting, no cooking.

Negatives:

Delivered food tastes like cardboard and more expensive than making your own.

How it works:

Calorie control.

The Scarsdale Diet

Positives:

Some may consider the fact that this diet encourages no exercise as a positive.

Negatives:

It is a true VLED, and not a long term plan.

How it works:

Calorie restriction and water loss.

Slim Fast

Positives:

Not as expensive as similar plans.

Negatives:

Nothing beats real food. Boring.

How it works:

Calorie restriction via shakes for breakfast and lunch.

Weight Watchers

Positives:

Good support with meetings and neato magnets and pins for prizes!

Negatives:

Group weigh-ins. Need to be part of a group to understand their rhetoric.

How it works:

Calorie restriction portion control using point system.

Cabbage Soup

Positives:

If you like cabbage soup, this is the one for you!

Negatives:

Nutritionally inadequate, boring, and will give you gas and diarrhea.

How it works:

Calorie restriction to the max!

Optifast

Positives:

Quick weight loss.

Negatives:

No chewing i.e. no food – weight comes back like a son-of-a-gun if you do not transition correctly.

How it works:

Doctor supervised calorie restriction liquid fast.

Overeaters Anonymous

Positives:

Good support with meetings and phone.

Negatives:

It is a 12 step program like AA; however, you cannot quit foods entirely (like you can alcohol).

How it works:

Emotional control over food and portion control.

Bob Greene Diet Plan

Positives:

Focuses on behaviors and motivation. No food restrictions.

Negatives:

Most people would need a personal in-home chef and personal trainer, like Oprah had with Mr. Greene.

How it works:

Lots of exercise and portion control.

The Slow Food Diet Plan

Positives:

No calorie counting, all organic food (for what that is worth).

Negatives:

Very expensive. Difficult to prepare meals. Preachy.

How it works:

It is so expensive, you cannot afford to eat a lot, therefore caloric restriction.

The Makers Plan

Positives:

No portion control (? positive).

Negatives:

Unusual requirements on showering, chlorine, etc. I was not aware GOD had an eating plan. If he did, I would not have written this book and I would have endorsed his to the fullest.

How it works:

Subtle caloric restriction.

The Sonoma Diet

Positives:

Good foods!

Negatives:

Takes some work so it is time consuming. Being a professional chef is also of great benefit.

How it works:

Caloric restriction by portion control.

Appendix III

The Z Diet and Holidays, Parties, and Office Goodies

How to survive the occasional party:
- Eat before the event
    - High protein/fruit/vegetables 30 min before the event
- Never go to a party hungry
    - Take a lower calorie/low fat dessert or dish to the party
    - Review How to shop and read labels
- Don't ignore the temptation, just be wise in your amounts
    - Once piece of cake, not five!
    - Make Better Bad Choices!

Exercise during holidays
- Don't skip on exercise just due to the time of year

- Don't think you will "make up" later for missing your workout
- Train harder during the holidays!
  - Increase your intensity and amounts
- "prepare" your body for food storage
  - Train REALLY hard the days immediately before and after the **Events, Parties, and the day of celebration**

Events, Parties, and the day of celebration

- Take a scheduled or prescription break in your diet plan
  - Train REALLY hard the days immediately before and after the **Events, Parties, and the day of celebration**
- Eat a lower carbohydrate diet the days preceding and following the event
  - Consider intermittent fasting
- Stay away from the scale!
  - Water weight vs. actual fat weight
- Don't ignore the temptation, just be wise in your amounts
  - Once piece of cake, not five!
  - Make Better Bad Choices!
- For the REALLY anal:
  - Bring your own food!

How to survive the office treats:

- When Scheduled, schedule!
  - Bring your own food!

Appendix IV

Contact Information

If you are interested in a personal consult I can be contacted at the following numbers and address:

Walk In Weight Loss

Attn: Dr. Warren Willey

134 Chubbuck Rd.

Chubbuck, Idaho 83202

Office Phone: 208.237.7911

Office Fax: 208.237.3450

Web Site: www.walkinweightloss.com and www.eatright4u.com

Email: warren@walkinweightloss.com

If you are interested in an on-line consult please visit: http://www.eatright4u.com/fatlosseconsult.html

eConsultations provided by Dr. Willey are for informational purposes only. Interventions and suggestions fall in the realm of weight loss, lean mass gain, and attainment of body goals. Medical diagnosis, intervention, and/or treatment including prescrip-

tions WILL NOT be provided online. If you desire or need such services or advice, you are welcome to see Dr. Willey in person at his clinic.

My personal email address is: docjww@yahoo.com

To order books, fat measuring devices, and DVDs go to http://www.eatright4u.com/store.html

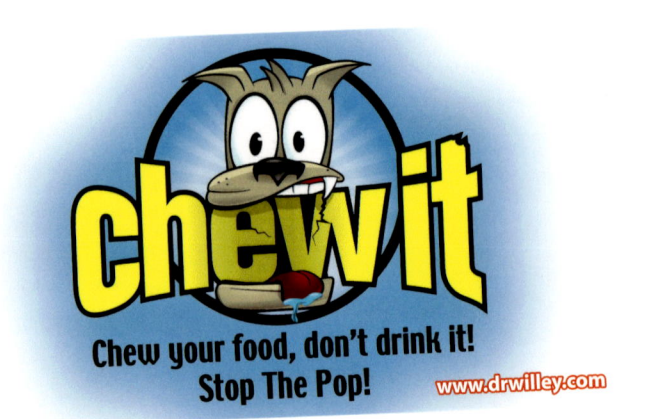

Dr. Willey's Bio

Dr. Warren Willey is the Medical Director of a medical weight loss center and primary care office in southeast Idaho. He uses a unique approach to patient care by offering preventative medical intervention by helping people to obtain optimal health and fitness through elite nutritional programs, diet strategies, and exercise programs. He is a Board Certified Osteopathic Physician, and did his postgraduate training at The Mayo Clinic. He is a founding diplomat of the American Board of Holistic medicine and a diplomat with The America Board of Family Medicine, The America Board Urgent Care Medicine and The American Board of Bariatric Medicine.

Dr. Willey is highly sought after, dynamic speaker and does healthy living and weight loss presentations around the country. Dr. Willey is an established author having written a medical textbook and **What Does Your Doctor Look Like Naked**? Your guide To Optimum Health, released in 2003. This book has helped thousands of people lose weight and obtain and then maintain optimal health. One of his books, **Better Than Steroids**!, is sold internationally as it is the most concise summary of what you need to know to get that ultimate physique! He also writes for a number periodicals and web sites. He has 25 years experience with exercise development and nutritional intervention.